Your Supervised Practicum and Internship

FIELD RESOURCES FOR TURNING THEORY INTO ACTION

Your Supervised Practicum and Internship

FIELD RESOURCES FOR TURNING THEORY INTO ACTION

LORI A. RUSSELL-CHAPIN
Bradley University

ALLEN E. IVEY
University of Massachusetts, Amherst (Emeritus)
President, Microtraining Associates, Inc.

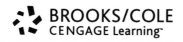

BROOKS/COLE
CENGAGE Learning™

Australia • Brazil • Japan • Korea • Mexico • Singapore • Spain • United Kingdom • United States

BROOKS/COLE
CENGAGE Learning

Your Surpervised Practicum and Internship: Field Resources for Turning Theory into Action
Lori A. Russell-Chapin, Allen E. Ivey

Executive Editor: Lisa Gebo

Assistant Editor: Alma Dea Michelena

Editorial Assistant: Sheila Walsh

Technology Project Manager: Barry Connolly

Marketing Manager: Caroline Concilla

Marketing Assistant: Mary Ho

Advertising Project Manager: Tami Strang

Project Manager, Editorial Production:
 Katy German

Print/Media Buyer: Rebecca Cross

Permissions Editor: Sommy Ko

Production Service: UG / GGS Information
 Services, Inc.

Copy Editor: Jennifer D'Inezo

Cover Designer: Roger Knox

Cover Image: Lois Grady

For product information and technology assistance, contact us at
Cengage Learning Customer & Sales Support, 1-800-354-9706

For permission to use material from this text or product,
submit all requests online at **www.cengage.com/permissions**
Further permissions questions can be emailed to
permissionrequest@cengage.com

Library of Congress Control Number: 2003107200

ISBN-13: 978-0-534-60615-2

ISBN-10: 0-534-60615-6

Brooks/Cole
10 Davis Drive
Belmont, CA 94002
USA

Cengage Learning is a leading provider of customized learning solutions with office locations around the globe, including Singapore, the United Kingdom, Australia, Mexico, Brazil, and Japan. Locate your local office at **international.cengage.com/region**

Cengage Learning products are represented in Canada by Nelson Education, Ltd.

For your course and learning solutions, visit **academic.cengage.com**

Purchase any of our products at your local college store or at our preferred online store **www.ichapters.com**

Printed in the United States of America
  4 5 6 7 8   14 13 12 11 10

ED256

Contents

Preface   *xiii*
About the Authors   *xxiii*

Section One

GETTING STARTED: YOU, SUPERVISION, AND THE SETTINGS   1

Chapter 1

Turning Theory into Practice: Abilities Needed to Grow   2

Overview   3
Goals   3
Key Concepts: Needed Abilities for a Successful Field Experience   3
   Risk Taking   4
   Practical Reflection 1: Identifying Fears and Concerns   4
   Goal Setting and Areas for Growth and Development   5
   Practical Reflection 2: Establishing Goals   6
   Feedback   6
   Practical Reflection 3: Corrective Feedback   7
   Respect   7
   Power   8
   Practical Reflection 4: Power Differentials   9
   Multicultural Issues   9
   Practical Reflection 5: Multicultural Concerns   10
   Positive Resources and Personal Strengths   10
   Practical Reflection 6: Emphasizing Your Personal Strengths   11
   Other Key Issues for the Success of Your
     Field Experience, Practicum, and Internship   11
   *Practical Reflection 7: Analyzing Past Transference
    and Countertransference Issues*   14

v

Summary and Personal Integration   15
    Practical Reflection 8: Integration   15

Chapter 2

Listening to Tapes and Analyzing Cases: Microcounseling Supervision   17

Overview   18
Goals   18
Key Concepts: Microcounseling Supervision   18
The Three Components of Microcounseling Supervision   20
    Reviewing Microcounseling Skills With Intention   20
    Practical Reflection 1: Reviewing Skills With Intention   21
    Classifying Skills With Mastery   21
    Practical Reflection 2: Classifying Skills With Mastery   22
    Processing Supervisory Needs   26
Supervisory Process   28
    Practical Reflection 3: Summarizing and Processing Skills   28
Uses of the CIRF   28
    Case Presentation   29
    Practical Reflection and Self-Assessment 4: Establishing Your
        Counseling Skills Baseline   30
    Practical Reflection 5: Understanding Microcounseling Supervision   30
Summary and Personal Integration   31
    Practical Reflection 6: Integration   31
Resource A: Glossary of CIRF Skills   33
Resource B: Microskill Classification: Transcript of Rachel and Lori   38
Resource C: Counseling Interview Rating Form   41
Resource D: Counseling Interview Rating Form   43
Resource E: Counseling Interview Rating Form   46

Chapter 3

Becoming Effective as a Supervisee: The Influence of Placement Setting   48

Overview   49
Goals   49
Key Concepts: You and Supervision   49
Determining Which Supervision Style Works Best for You   50
    Developmental Styles of Supervision   50
    Practical Reflection 1: The Best Fit Supervisory Styles   52
    Practical Reflection 2: Preferred Maturity Dimensions   52
    Practical Reflection 3: Current Supervisory Expectations   52
You and Your Supervision Setting   53
    School Settings   53
    Primary, Middle, and High Schools   53

The Case of Stephen
    Practical Reflection 4: School Counseling Supervisory Needs   59
    Colleges and Universities   59
    Community Agencies   61
    Private Practice   64
    Hospital-Based Treatment Programs   66
    Practical Reflection 5: Influences of Field Experience Settings   68
Collecting and Sharing Needed Information   68
    Practical Reflection 6: Student Practicum/Internship Agreement   69
Evaluation of Your Work in the Placement Setting   70
    Practical Reflection 7: Evaluation Concerns   71
Summary and Personal Integration   71
    Practical Reflection 8: Integration   72
Resource F: Supervisory Styles Inventory   73
Resource G: Author's Quantification of CIRF of the Case of Stephen   75
Resource H: Student Practicum/Internship Agreement   78
Resource I: Practicum/Internship Contract   79
Resource J: Weekly Log Sheet   81
Resource K: Client Informed Consent Form   82
Resource L: Client Release Form   83
Resource M: Site Supervisor's Evaluation of Student
   Counselor's Performance   84

Chapter 4

Continuing Self-Improvement: Major Supervision Model Categories   87

Overview   88
Goals   88
Key Concepts: Finding the Supervision Match for You   88
Developmental Models of Supervision   89
    Practical Reflection 1: Developmental Model Growth Areas   90
Integrated Models of Supervision   90
    Practical Reflection 2: Role and Focus Needs   91
Theory-Specific Supervision Models   92
    Practical Reflection 3: Theoretical Orientation   92
A Supervision Videotaping Method: Interpersonal Process Recall   93
    Practical Reflection 4: Needed IPR Questions   94
Supervision and the Case of Rachel   94
    Developmental Supervision and the Case of Rachel   94
    Integrated Supervision and the Case of Rachel   95
    Theoretically Oriented Supervision and the Case of Rachel   95
    Practical Reflection 5: Your Favorite Supervision Model   96
    Practical Reflection 6: You and Your Supervision Perceptions   96
Summary and Personal Integration   97
    Practical Reflection 7: Integration   97

Resource N: Microcounseling Skills Used in Different
    Theoretical Approaches   99
Resource O: Supervisee Perception of Supervision   100

Chapter 5

Conceptualizing the Client: Diagnosis and Related Issues   103

Overview   104
Goals   104
Key Concepts: Client Case Conceptualization and the Investigative
    Nature of Counseling   104
    Confidentiality   105
    Humble Guest   105
    Cautiousness   106
Case Conceptualization Methods   107
    Using the Interview Stages to Conceptualize Cases   107
    Practical Reflection 1: Stages of the Interview   108
    Adding the DSM-IV-TR to the Case Conceptualization   108
Diagnosis Using the DSM-IV-TR   109
    DSM-IV-TR Axis I—Clinical Syndromes and Other Conditions
        That May Be a Focus of Clinical Attention   109
    DSM-IV-TR Axis II—Personality Disorders and Mental
        Retardation   110
    DSM-IV-TR Axis III—General Medical Concerns   111
    DSM-IV-TR Axis IV—Psychosocial and Environmental
        Problems   112
    DSM-IV-TR Axis V—Global Assessment of Functioning   112
    Practical Reflection 2: DSM-IV-TR Strategy and
        Conceptualization   113
Developmental Assessment   113
    Practical Reflection 3: Your Preferred Developmental
        Orientation Style   116
Goals and Treatment Plans   116
Case Presentation Guidelines   117
    Narrative Case Presentation About Rachel   117
    Practical Reflection 4: Case Presentation Additions   119
The Case of Rachel: Case Conceptualization With the Stages of the Interview,
    Clinical Diagnosis, and Developmental Assessment   120
    Stages of the Interview   120
    DSM-IV-TR Diagnosis   120
    Developmental Assessment   121
    Goals and Treatment for Rachel   121
Summary and Personal Integration   122
    Practical Reflection 5: Integration   123
Resource P: Microskills Hierarchy   124
Resource Q: Case Presentation Outline Guide   125

Section Two

KNOWLEDGE NEEDED TO GROW: ISSUES IN PROFESSIONAL PRACTICE   127

Chapter 6

Becoming a Culturally Competent Helping Professional: Appreciation of Diversity   128

Overview   129
Goals   129
Key Concepts: A Continuum for Multicultural
    Development   129
Cross-Cultural Dimensions in Counseling   130
    Family Context   130
    Social Systems Context   130
    Demographic Context   130
    *Practical Reflection 1: Examining Your Cultural Beliefs
        About Helping*   131
    Status Context   131
    Life Experience Context   131
You and Multicultural Competence   131
    Attitudes and Beliefs Guidelines   132
    *Practical Reflection 2: Influential Experiences Influencing Your
        Cultural Identity*   133
    Knowledge Guidelines   133
    Practical Reflection 3: Stereotype Development   134
    *Practical Reflection 4: Proactive Experiences in
        Multicultural Development*   135
    Skill Guidelines   135
    Models of Racial Identity Development   135
    Practical Reflection 5: Racial Identity Development   137
    An Example Approach for Enhancing Diversity Appreciation:
        A Diversity Simulation   137
    Practical Reflection 6: Albatrossian Simulation   139
Example Interview: The Case of Darryl   140
    The Case of Darryl   140
    The Case of Darryl: A Multicultural Perspective   146
    Practical Reflection 7: Response to the Case of Darryl   146
Summary and Personal Integration   147
    Practical Reflection 8: Integration   147
Resource R: Counseling Interview Rating Form   149
*Resource S: Author's Quantification of CIRF Summarization and Processing
    Skills of the Case of Darryl*   151
Resource T: The Case of Darryl with Skill Identification   155

Chapter 7
Working With Ethics, Laws, and Professionalism: Best Practice Standards   161

Overview   162
Goals   162
Key Concepts: Standards of Care   162
Ethics and Ethical Behaviors   164
    Practical Reflection 1: Ethical Behavior   165
Code of Ethics   165
    *Practical Reflection 2: Comprehending Your Profession's
      Code of Ethics*   166
Case Notes, Record Keeping, and HIPAA Information   166
    *Practical Reflection 3: Writing Concise Case Notes Focusing
      on HIPAA Compliance*   168
The Process of Referring Clients to Other Practitioners   168
    Practical Reflection 4: The Referral Process   169
Utilizing Case Law   169
    Confidentiality and Duty to Warn   169
    Privileged Communication   170
    Practical Reflection 5: Understanding Case Law   171
Professionalism and Professional Behaviors   171
    *Practical Reflection 6: Recognizing Professional
      Behaviors*   172
Professional Organizations   172
Ethical and Professional Behaviors: The Case of Darryl   173
Summary and Personal Integration   173
    Practical Reflection 7: Dilemmas in the Case of Darryl   174
    Practical Reflection 8: Integration   174
*Resource U: Web Addresses for Professional Organizations
  and Codes of Ethics*   176
Resource V: ACA Code of Ethics and Standards of Practice   177

Chapter 8
Counseling Research Outcomes: Discovering What Works   207

Overview   208
Goals   208
Key Concepts: Practicing Evidence-Based Counseling   208
A Brief History of Counseling Effectiveness and Change   209
    Practical Reflection 1: Beginning to Practice Outcome Research   210
Types of Outcome Research   210
    Descriptive Research   211
    Quantitative Designs   211
    Program, Client, Counselor, and Supervision Evaluations   212
    Meta-Analysis   213

Qualitative Designs   213
Practical Reflection 2: Selecting the Most Efficient Research Type for You   214
Research Practitioner Models   214
Scientist/Practitioner Model   214
Practical Reflection 3: Clarifying Your Strengths and Liabilities   215
Teacher/Scholar Model   215
Practical Reflection 4: Choosing Your Best Fit Scholarly Function   216
Summary and Personal Integration   216
Practical Reflection 5: Integration   217
Resource W: Indirect Evidence: Methods for Evaluating the Presence of Nontherapy Explanations   219

Chapter 9

Staying Well: Guidelines for Responsible Living   *220*

Overview   221
Goals   221
Key Concepts: A Balanced Lifestyle With Proportion, Not Equity   221
Rules for Responsible Living   222
Practical Reflection 1: Clarifying Your Values   223
Practical Reflection 2: Assessing Your Locus of Control   224
Physical Health   224
Emotional Well-Being   225
Intellectual Enrichment   225
Life Work Satisfaction   225
Social Effectiveness   225
Practical Reflection 3: Your Lifestyle Assessment Score   226
Spiritual Awareness   226
Practical Reflection 4: Wellness and You: Setting Personal Goals   227
Practical Reflection 5: The Case of Darryl and Counselor Wellness   228
Summary and Personal Integration   228
Practical Reflection 6: Integration   228
Resource X: Rotter's Locus of Control Scale   230
Resource Y: The Lifestyle Assessment Survey, Form C   234

Chapter 10

Becoming a Professional Helper: Advocacy for Clients, Self, and the Profession   *237*

Overview   238
Goals   238
Key Concepts: Advocacy and Its Relationship to the Ten Essential Principles for Helping Professionals   238
Advocacy for the Client   238

Advocacy for Self   239
Advocacy for the Profession   240
    Practical Reflection 1: Your Advocacy Efforts   240
Ten Essential Chapter Principles for Helping Professionals   240
    1. Transferable Skills, Abilities, and Principles   240
    Practical Reflection 2: Looking Back and Comparing Feelings   241
    2. Creative Interchanges Through Core Interviewing Skills   241
    3. The Path of Right Action   242
    4. Flexibility in Growth   242
    5. Telling the Entire Story   242
    6. Universal Communication Skills   242
    7. Risk Management and the World of Counseling   243
    8. Evidence-Based Best Practice   243
    9. Helping Self and Others   244
    Practical Reflection 3: Writing New Goals for Your Professional Life   244
    10. Where Am I Now and Where Do I Need to Go?   245
Summary and Personal Integration   246
    Practical Reflection 4: Integration and Lessons Learned   246
Resource Z: Chi Sigma Iota Advocacy Themes   247

***Index of Names*   249**

***Index of Subjects*   253**

Preface

BEFORE YOU START

We welcome you to one of the most exciting and, certainly most personally involving, courses in the helping field. Working with clients, their families, and the community is what it is all about. The field experience, practicum, or internship all give you a chance to show what you can do. It is a place you can test out those theories and see if they really work.

Feedback is said to be the breakfast of champions. We recommend that you use the many resources available to you to gain as much information about yourself and your work as you possibly can. We provide a large number of resources in this book. But, seek feedback from your colleagues and supervisors. Having others look at your work can be challenging, but it is here that you can grow the most. We suggest that you use your practicum, internship, or field experience as a foundation for your entire professional life. It is vital that you listen carefully to clients so that you can help them grow; you, too, will grow if you listen equally carefully to those supporting your development.

Each of us would like to share some thoughts about how to use this book and the importance of the field experience, internship and practicum.

ALLEN

I'll just share one personal story as we begin. My first practical experience in counseling was an intern in the counseling center at Tufts University under the wise guidance of Alvin Schmidt, director. I certainly was inexperienced in a professional role and felt more than a bit awkward. How would I survive my first interview?

Luckily for me, Schmidt had a ready smile and was completely supportive and confident that I would be up to the job, even though he had no evidence for that fact. That first interview was neither particularly good, nor particularly bad, but reviewing it with him made an immediate difference. I learned that it was okay to make mistakes and that I could learn and grow from them. I learned from Alvin Schmidt, the person, that relationship is key and the nature of the person who is the counselor or therapist is as important as book knowledge. Not all of you will have the patient mentor that I enjoyed, but there is something to learn from the feedback offered by all supervisors.

Theory is vital, but it is people like you and me that take it into practice. Growing as a person and as a therapist is one of the goals of this text. We are going to share some ideas, but it is you who will use some of them and make them work.

Schmidt also taught me something the books at that time did not cover. I found it critical that I learn the ways of his agency, the counseling center, as quickly as possible. Forms, reports, and ethical standards were an important part of the job. I also discovered it was important to meet and know faculty members and administrators in the Tufts community. We tend to learn counseling and therapy in isolation, but it is practiced in a community context. If we are to be effective, we need to be community members and tailor our work to community needs.

Multicultural issues are an important part of the context of counseling. Lori and I define culture broadly to include race and ethnicity, gender, socioeconomic status, sexual orientation, ability/disability, age, spirituality, and other relevant factors such as language (bilingual ability is an asset not a liability) or experience of trauma (a person who experienced rape, AIDS, cancer, loss of parent, or war has entered a special culture). Each community agency exists within a cultural setting, unique to itself. I suggest that you spend some time going beyond the immediate agency setting and learning about the community within which you work.

Let us now turn to what we have to share with you. We've both enjoyed and profited from being supervised and supervising others. After you have completed work with this text, we'd enjoy hearing from you and obtaining your feedback. You can contact me at ivey@srnet.com. Please note the feedback form at the close of this book. It has been a delight to work with Lori on this book. She'll tell you below some of the origins of the ideas we present and how they might be helpful to you.

Keep in touch and let us grow together. We welcome your feedback and suggestions letting us know how you experienced this book.

LORI

I'd like to share with you how this text got started. I have been teaching graduate-level practicum and internship counseling courses for the past

15 years. These field experience courses are my very favorite classes, as I have the great pleasure of watching all of you, the novice counseling trainees, transform into skilled helping professionals. It is a time of immense personal changes and growth.

The difficulty of this class for me was that I have never found the exact textbook that could assist you and me through this exciting but scary experience. I often used supplemental texts and individual monographs, but again there was no book that focused on all the essential areas of the field experience.

As I began creating many of my own tools, I became aware that so much of what I believe about the helping profession came from the work of Dr. Allen Ivey. I bravely decided to ask Dr. Ivey and his wife, Dr. Mary Bradford Ivey, to travel to Bradley University to be guest speakers at one of our alumni events. That was the beginning of this textbook, as Allen and I began to brainstorm enthusiastically about the needs of a field experience book that would integrate all aspects of the field experience from developmental concerns to ethics to conceptualization to supervision!

The Need for This Text: My First Client Memory

It was my first day as a new counselor working in a mental health clinic in western United States. I was 25 years old, and I was ready! Now I could truly make a difference in the world! Trying to remember all the skills I was supposed to do was intimidating, but I felt confident. I had dressed professionally. I still remember what I was wearing, a brown shirtdress and matching shoes! I arrived early to work and I was just waiting patiently.

Finally it was 9 o'clock in the morning. My client's intake form had been placed in her file. In walked Rachel. She was a tall woman and from her information, she was 71 years old. Before I could say "hello," before I could attempt to talk about confidentiality, and before I could speak of the counseling process, Rachel began to pace in the room and silently stare at me. She would not sit down in any of the available chairs in my office. She continued to walk around the office, carefully observing me from top to bottom. Finally Rachel snorted, "Honey, what could you possibly have to offer me? You are a child with very little life experience, and you will never be able to help or understand my problems!"

I was stunned, of course. I do remember thinking, did any of my professors or supervisors tell me what to do when this happens? I decided to be silent, not as an intentional skill, but because I did not know what else to do! Then I recalled some concept called resistance. I decided to just go with it. Rachel continued to rant, and finally there was a small lull, so I responded, "Rachel, you are probably correct. I have not lived as long as you, and I don't have as much life experience as you. All I can do is listen to you and see if a counseling relationship develops. How does that sound to you?" Fortunately for Rachel and me, that intentional response was one that worked! That was 25 years ago, and I remember it like yesterday.

For You, the Student

Your Supervised Practicum and Internship: Field Resources For Turning Theory into Action will be about you and your first clients, too. The primary focus of this book is to offer you a comprehensive foundation and guide for your practicum and internship field experiences. It will be about your personal journey as a student as you progress and evolve through the final aspects of your graduate education.

Praxis: The Central Goal of this Book. The teaching philosophy of the entire book uses the concept of *praxis*, or turning theory into practice. Utilizing this concept, you will be able to integrate all aspects of the field experience through practical application of the three case studies presented, exercises, practical reflections, and individual assessments.

Further to assist praxis, A Summary List of Resources that correspond to each chapter is provided. These 26 unique resources, labeled from Resource A to Resource Z, will assist you in your practicum and internship. All of these features will make your transition from counseling theory to counseling practice much easier and smoother. Some of these forms you will use as they are; others you will want to shape and adapt, in consultation with your instructor and/or supervisor, to fit your own field placement setting.

What really counts, of course, is you, your motivation, and your willingness to learn. At the same time, you also have a lot to share with clients, colleagues, and supervisors. We wish you well on this important journey as you personally turn theory into practice.

For You, the Instructor. If you would like your students to have access to InfoTrac® College Edition, contact your local Wadsworth/Brooks/ Cole representative prior to placing your book order so that you can be sure to request the special ISBN that will offer InfoTrac® College Edition with each new copy of the book. If you are an instructor of higher education and have adopted this new textbook, a free CD-ROM is available upon request! Just contact your Wadsworth/Brooks/Cole Representative, and they in turn will call the Marketing Assistant for the Helping Professions, with your mailing address. That person will place the order for you through Microtraining Associates. I use the CD in my classes, and the students thoroughly enjoy this interactive method of learning Microcounseling Supervision and the microcounseling skills. There is also a video on Microcounseling Supervision available from Microtraining. Contact them at 1-888-505-5576 or www.emicrotraining.com.

BOOK FEATURES

First, and foremost, this book is filled with resources to guide you through your field experience. Each chapter has practical reflections and examples of resources you can utilize from instruments assessing your supervision style to forms to assist you in analyzing your interviewing skills. Although we have presented the chapters in a special order, some of you may prefer to arrange the chapters in an order that may meet your teaching and learning specifications better. The chapters can stand alone, so be sure to use the text in the manner best suited your needs.

The book has been developed in two sections. Section One, Getting Started: You, Supervision, and the Settings, has five chapters that address vital areas of supervision, the need for feedback, and the essentials of client conceptualization, diagnosis, and treatment. You will learn more about Rachel throughout Section One; Rachel and her story will be the first of the three case studies presented. The second case study presented in Section One is about Stephen, an 11-year-old boy whose father committed suicide. I worked with Stephen in a school setting when he was referred to me because his grades were falling and he was increasingly isolating himself from friends and family.

Section Two, Knowledge Needed to Grow: Issues in Professional Practice, has five chapters, and in these chapters you will concentrate on areas that concern all helping professionals such as multicultural competencies and ethics and the law. Additionally, Section Two helps you to learn about the importance of outcome-based research on supervision, evaluation of your counseling skills, and focusing on your own well-being as a helping professional.

The third case study you will work with in Section Two is about a young man named Darryl. He was referred to me years later in my counseling career, because he was having difficulty keeping his job, his marriage was failing, and he stated that he just could not keep it together. By that time I was teaching in a university setting and counseling in a private practice one day a week. I had just terminated with one client, so an opening was available.

Once again, I was prepared to conduct an initial intake session, when Darryl took one look at me and began talking in tongues. I had little idea as what to do, so I listened respectfully. When Darryl was finished, he curled up into a fetal position on my floor. Once more, I thought, did any of my professors prepare me for this?! One of my first instincts was to call security for help, but I calmed myself down and moved to the floor with him! Darryl remained in that dissociative position for 45 minutes.

When he finally sat up, I was still sitting on the floor with him. He inquired about the session, and I told him what I observed. We processed our first session. Darryl asked to leave but wanted to set up another appointment! I set up another appointment for him, and then I called my supervisor for an appointment that was sooner than a week away! You will learn more about Darryl throughout Section Two.

Chapter Topics

Each chapter topic is critical to your success in field experience and supervision. The material can have a direct and practical application to your practicum and internship. In Chapter 1, "Turning Theory Into Practice: Abilities Needed to Grow," you are introduced to seven practical abilities necessary for a successful field experience. These abilities allow you as a novice helping professional to address fears and concerns of beginning a field experience. The chapter allows you to provide a frank discussion of risk taking, goal setting, feedback, respect, power, multicultural issues, strengths, and available resources.

Chapter 2, "Listening to Tapes and Analyzing Cases: Microcounseling Supervision," provides a basic supervision model that teaches you a general vocabulary for reviewing the fundamental interviewing skills with intention, classifying those same skills with mastery, and summarizing your counseling interview style with an individualized supervision session. The Microcounseling Supervision Model teaches you the needed information to actively listen to counseling tapes and provide corrective feedback needed to grow in your field experience.

Chapter 3, "Becoming Effective as a Supervisee: The Influence of Placement Setting," introduces you to dimensions of effective supervision and the influences that your chosen placement setting may have on your field experiences.

In Chapter 4, "Continuing Self-Improvement: Major Categories of Supervision Models," you are introduced to additional supervision models that will help you continue to grow in your field experience. The final chapter in Section One is Chapter 5, "Conceptualizing the Client: Diagnosis and Related Issues." This chapter assists you in conceptualizing your client's case and diagnosing using the DSM-IV-TR, if necessary.

There are five chapters in Section Two, Knowledge Needed to Grow. Chapter 6, "Becoming a Culturally Competent Helping Professional: Appreciation of Diversity," focuses on issues surrounding diversity and the manner in which your racial identity has developed.

In Chapter 7, "Working With Ethics, Laws, and Professionalism: Best Practice Standards," ethics are differentiated from professionalism, and landmark case laws are presented. The newly mandated HIPPA requirements are discussed as well. Chapter 8, "Counseling Research Outcomes: Discovering What Works," outlines the effectiveness of counseling with outcome research.

The final two chapters are designed to help bring closure to your capstone experience. Chapter 9, "Staying Well: Guidelines for Responsible Living," helps you to assess your own personal wellness and any areas of impairment. Chapter 10, "Becoming a Professional Helper: Advocating for Clients, Self and the Profession," assists you in evaluating your progress to date and emphasizes the importance of advocacy for yourself and the counseling profession.

A Guide

Please use this book as a resource guide to assist you on the adventures of becoming a skilled helping professional. Your efforts will not go unnoticed. Your skill level will increase, and you will be rewarded with added confidence, wisdom, and continued curiosity about counseling and personal growth! Allen and I will assist you through this exciting journey! The following poem by Rumi sets the stage perfectly for your challenges and growth to come.

The Guest House

This being human is a guest house.
Every morning is a new arrival.
A joy, a depression, a meanness,
some momentary awareness comes
as an unexpected visitor.

Welcome and entertain them all!
Even if they're a crowd of sorrows,
who violently sweep your house
empty of its furniture,
still, treat each guest honorably.
He may be clearing you out
for some new delight.

The dark thought, the shame, the malice,
meet them at the door laughing,
and invite them in.

Be grateful for whoever comes,
because each has been sent
as a guide from beyond.

Acknowledgments

This book has been a labor of love. Being a member of the helping profession is an avocation for me! As I have developed and grown as a person and clinician, it has been fun to share many of my observations and ideas with others in the profession. I would like to thank the following persons who assisted me by reviewing this book in its manuscript form: John A. Casey, California State University, Bakersfield; Donna Kennealley, University of South Dakota; Jeff Schrenzel, Western New England College; Mary Davidson, Columbia-Greene Community College; Carol W. Adler, Ohio University, Athens; Barbara H. Cohen, California State University, Long Beach; Kenneth B. Johnson, Amberton University; Robert A. Silverberg, Kent State University; LeeAnn M. Eschbach, University of Scranton.

But even more important are the people who have influenced me by their generosity, compassion, and dedication not only to the field of counseling but to life in general. This book is dedicated to all those people in my life who are mentors and role models to me. These people epitomize the concept of "richly living" by taking risks and generating new options.

THANK YOU TO

My children, Elissa and Jaimeson, who keep me focused on the moment

My client, Christine, who lost her life but faced her fears

Our editor, Lisa, whose wisdom and clarity has been so appreciated

My husband, Ted, whose love and friendship have provided me with support but challenged me toward mastery

My mentor, Allen Ivey, who has inspired me and countless others to be passionate about the counseling field

My mother, Helen, who models for me that life is about constant growth

My sister, Debi, who is recovering from a stroke and whose courage and desire for life is contagious

My students and my GA, Victoria, whose dedicated quest for knowledge and skills keeps the counseling profession strong and progressive. If any of you need to contact me, my email address is lar@bradley.edu.

LORI

Reference

Barks, C. (1995). *The Essential Rumi*. San Francisco: HarperCollins. Reprinted by HarperCollins Publishers, Inc.

SUMMARY LIST OF RESOURCES

Resource A: Glossary of Counseling Interview Rating Form Skills (CIRF)—Reviewing Skills With Intention

Resource B: Author's Microskill Classifications of the Case of Rachel—Classifying Skills With Mastery

Resource C: Blank Counseling Interview Rating Form—Student's Use for Summarization and Quantification of the Case of Rachel

Resource D: Author's Quantification of CIRF—Summarizing and Processing Skills

Resource E: Blank CIRF—Establishing Personal Baseline of Counseling Skills

Resource F: Supervisory Style Inventory

Resource G: Author's CIRF Quantification of the Case of Stephen

Resource H: Student Practicum/Internship Agreement

Resource I: Practicum/Internship Contract—University and Site

Resource J: Weekly Log Sheet

Resource K: Client Informed Consent Form

Resource L: Client Release Form

Resource M: Site Supervisor Evaluation of Student Counselor's Performance

Resource N: Microcounseling Skills Used in Differing Theoretical Approaches

Resource O: Supervisee Perception of Supervision

Resource P: Microskills Hierarchy

Resource Q: Case Presentation Outline Guide

Resource R: Blank CIRF

Resource S: Author's Quantification of CIRF—Summarization and Processing Skills of the Case of Darryl

Resource T: Script of the Case of Darryl With Skill Identification

Resource U: Web Addresses of Codes of Ethics

Resource V: ACA Code of Ethics

Resource W: Indirect Evidence of Counseling Change

Resource X: Rotter's Locus of Control Scale

Resource Y: Lifestyle Assessment Survey

Resource Z: Chi Sigma Iota Advocacy Themes

About the Authors

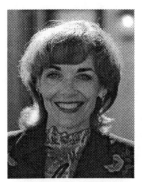

Dr. Lori Russell-Chapin was the Chair of the Counseling program for eleven years at Bradley University in Illinois. Currently, she is the Associate Dean of the College of Education and Health Sciences. Lori has worked as a clinical supervisor for many years, currently teaches the practicum and internship courses at Bradley University, and works in private practice. She is a Licensed Professional Clinical Counselor and a NBCC Approved Clinical Supervisor.

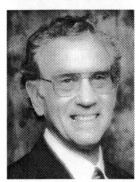

Dr. Allen E. Ivey is Distinguished University Professor (Emeritus), University of Massachusetts, Amherst. He is the president of Microtraining Associates, an educational publishing firm. Allen also serves on the Board of Directors of the National Institute for Multicultural Competence. Allen is author or coauthor of more than 30 books and 200 articles and chapters, translated into at least 16 languages. He is the originator of the microskills approach, basic to this book.

GETTING STARTED: YOU, SUPERVISION, AND THE SETTINGS

By the time you have completed Section one and the first five chapters, you may expect to:

- IDENTIFY YOUR STRENGTHS AND AREAS FOR IMPROVEMENTS TO ENSURE A SUCCESSFUL FIELD EXPERIENCE.
- PRESENT AND ANALYZE YOUR INTERVIEWS USING THE COUNSELING INTERVIEW RATING FORM AND MICROCOUNSELING SUPERVISION.
- UNDERSTAND THE DIMENSIONS OF EFFECTIVE SUPERVISION AND THE INFLUENCE YOUR PLACEMENT SETTING MAY HAVE ON SUPERVISION.
- LEARN ABOUT THE MAJOR SUPERVISION MODEL CATEGORIES.
- CONCEPTUALIZE YOUR CASE STUDIES USING THREE STRATEGIES: STAGES OF THE COUNSELING INTERVIEW, FORMAL DIAGNOSIS, AND DEVELOPMENTAL ASSESSMENT.

TURNING THEORY INTO PRACTICE: ABILITIES NEEDED TO GROW

▷ *The field experience takes courage—it facilitates growth most effectively if you allow yourself to become the person whom you truly are and want to be!*

OVERVIEW

GOALS

KEY CONCEPTS: NEEDED ABILITIES FOR A SUCCESSFUL FIELD EXPERIENCE
RISK TAKING
GOAL SETTING AND AREAS FOR GROWTH AND DEVELOPMENT
PRACTICAL REFLECTION 1: IDENTIFYING FEARS AND CONCERNS
PRACTICAL REFLECTION 2: ESTABLISHING GOALS
FEEDBACK
PRACTICAL REFLECTION 3: CORRECTIVE FEEDBACK
RESPECT
POWER

PRACTICAL REFLECTION 4: POWER DIFFERENTIALS
MULTICULTURAL ISSUES
PRACTICAL REFLECTION 5: MULTICULTURAL CONCERNS
POSITIVE RESOURCES AND PERSONAL STRENGTHS
PRACTICAL REFLECTION 6: EMPHASIZING YOUR PERSONAL STRENGTHS
OTHER KEY ISSUES FOR THE SUCCESS OF YOUR FIELD EXPERIENCE, PRACTICUM, AND INTERNSHIP
PRACTICAL REFLECTION 7: ANALYZING PAST TRANSFERENCE AND COUNTERTRANSFERENCE ISSUES

SUMMARY AND PERSONAL INTEGRATION
PRACTICAL REFLECTION 8: INTEGRATION

REFERENCES

OVERVIEW

Praxis: a teaching approach allowing theoretical material to integrate into practical and relevant skills and techniques.

This first chapter introduces you, the student, to the style and format of the entire book. Each chapter focuses on the concept of *praxis*, turning theory into practical skills. You will address seven abilities that you must practice to get the most out of your practicum, internship, and field experiences. Those necessary abilities address the following: risk taking, goal setting, feedback, respect, power, multicultural issues, and available resources.

GOALS

1. Delineate key aspects of the practicum and internship.
2. Focus on personal and professional issues that you will encounter frequently throughout your field experience.
3. List and analyze fears and concerns that may interfere with effectively completing your field experience.
4. Understand the dynamics of power throughout the field experience.
5. Identify at least four goals that need to be accomplished by the end of the field experience.

KEY CONCEPTS: NEEDED ABILITIES FOR A SUCCESSFUL FIELD EXPERIENCE

Educators are always looking for methods that assist you to "realize more and memorize less" (Albertson profiled in Bailey, 1986). The following sections emphasize just that. The presented ideas and reflections will guide, stimulate, and challenge you to integrate—not just memorize—what is needed to transform your theories into action. If you focus on each of the presented abilities, you will more easily realize and internalize what you need to gain from your practicum and internship.

There are seven essential abilities that will help you in getting started in your field experience. A successful beginning to your practicum and internship rests in your ability to take risks, set goals, and examine yourself openly. After classes and theory, you will find yourself facing clients. And your counseling practice will be reviewed by others—this itself is risk taking and requires a solid self-concept.

Feedback from others on your performance will prove invaluable, but is often challenging. Respect for yourself and others will enable you to hear supportive and corrective feedback. Power differentials underlie all classroom and agency work. Understanding how power issues play out will be helpful in your comfort in your field experiences. In addition, multicultural issues are present in all field experiences and your awareness and ability to consider these constantly is essential. Finally, discovering your available resources that can assist you in staying healthy is crucial to the overall success of your field experience.

Risk Taking

Risk taking: Assessing anxiety and fears and courageously changing old ways to facilitate new behaviors.

There is an old saying: you will get out of this course what you put into it! Practicum and internships are some of the most challenging, demanding, and essential courses of your graduate education. Not only must you "turn theory into practice," but each student must face individual fears and be willing to take risks as a budding counselor and as a valued peer supervisor to your classmates. This takes courage!

Carl Jung (1954) once inferred that one cannot be courageous unless one has been afraid and fearful! What a great statement. One of your first challenges in field experience is to face your fears and take calculated professional and personal risks. For example, in this course each of you will be required to demonstrate your counseling skills through audiotapes, videotapes, case presentations, and/or portfolio demonstrations. Showcasing your skills takes courage in itself. Insecurities are heightened and external locus of control is rampant. You want to do well in front of your professor and peers.

Practical Reflection 1: Identifying Fears and Concerns

Right now, begin your reflective journal for this chapter. First jot down your fears and concerns. These feelings and thoughts do not have to be shared with anyone. However, the more you are willing to share, the sooner you will begin to experience the concept of *universality*. Almost everyone in this class will have similar thoughts and feelings.

_____

_____

_____

_____

Try to remember that when others offer feedback about your tape, their comments do not reflect about you, the person, only about your skills. This is an important distinction. If this dichotomy is recognized, then you will desire the feedback even more, because it helps you to grow without the insecurities of approval.

Goal Setting and Areas for Growth and Development

One of the first things you must decide is what exactly you want out of this experience. Some students say they just want to complete the requirements with as little work as possible and jump through the necessary hoops. However, students who see their field experience as a powerful opportunity for growth will thrive! This kind of structured, organized, small group supervisory opportunity will not be as easily accessible again in your professional life. Seize this time with optimism and watch yourself change and grow as you never thought possible!

Decide what you want out of this course and set at least four tangible and measurable goals for yourself. Begin thinking about your prioritized goals for the field experience. Be sure to share with your classmates. Publicly stating your goals offers additional motivation and investment to achieve your desired outcomes. As you accomplish these goals, get into the habit of periodically setting new and additional goals.

The importance of goal setting seems to have the support of all helping professions. Not only does it strengthen the supervisee–supervisor relationship, but it offers specific and objective strategies to guide you in the learning process. You, your instructor, and your supervisor will want to set your goals during the first session. Be sure to set short- and long-term goals, reviewing and evaluating those goals throughout the field experience (Curtis, 2000).

For example, here are three sample goals that can help direct your field experience.

1. Even though I'm here a short time, I'd like to be able to become part of the total community of this service agency or school system. By the end of the first three weeks, I will have read the service directory with agency rules and guidelines, and I will introduce myself to three new co-workers each week.
2. I'd like to learn how to take corrective feedback positively. Too often, I fear hearing what others say. By the end of the first nine weeks, I will work with my supervisor to learn to use the feedback as a mechanism for change, not personal attacks.
3. To increase my skill confidence, I will practice one new counseling skill every week and discuss with my supervisor its effect and outcome.

Practical Reflection 2: Establishing Goals

Now begin your list of goals for this field experience. Courageously describe the outcome goals that you know you must learn to be a competent helping professional. These goals may have some similarity to others in this class, but your goals must be individual to meet your differing needs. List at least two short- and two long-term goals.

_____

_____

_____

_____

Feedback

Feedback: A communication skill offering perceptions, observations and information that the receiver may use to facilitate change.

As you think about your goals, review your strengths and liabilities. This is your chance to "pick the brains" of your university instructor, your on-site supervisors, and your classmates who each bring wisdom and expertise. Use this time constructively. Challenge yourself and your classmates to become the best helping professionals that you can.

The only way this challenge can take place, though, is to promise that constructive feedback will be offered. Constructive or corrective feedback is aimed at assisting you with changing some aspect of a particular skill.

Please remember, too, that feedback is best received when it has been asked for! Ask for it during your individual and class supervisory sessions. It must and should be your responsibility as a supervisee to request what you need and want. Do not leave that up to others. Very little will be gained if you leave your needs to others.

In addition, very little will be gained if you offer only positive and vague feedback to yourself and your peers. We often hear students make comments such as, "You were wonderful with that client. I am so impressed with your skills." Those words are nice to hear, but they will not help anyone grow and improve.

Please offer feedback that is constructive and very specific. In the next section, we will offer an example of one method of assisting you with constructive feedback using a form that can be used with videotapes or

Practical Reflection 3: Corrective Feedback

What corrective feedback do you need at this moment in your field experience? What specific issues for personal growth would be useful? In the past, how have you best received feedback? Ask for the assistance you need now.

_____

_____

_____

_____

live supervision. For now, though, remember the 80/20 rule of offering feedback. Make sure that 80 percent of the given feedback is positive and stated first, then the remaining 20 percent of constructive feedback can be heard. Demonstrating your skills is scary, as most of us do want approval from others. With the 80/20 method, you will receive needed support and have the courage to move forward.

Respect

Many of you have been with your professors and classmates for several courses. Some relationships have developed if you have taken risks and built necessary trust. If you are honest about your needs, fears, and concerns, the odds are that your fellow students will follow suit. To assert your thoughts, feelings, and ideas is basic assertiveness at its best. Showing mutual respect, the underpinnings of assertiveness, will allow your field experience to flourish and produce extremely beneficial results. Practice the belief that assertion breeds assertion, nonassertion breeds nonassertion, and aggression breeds aggression.

In your beginning theory class, you learned that empathy, unconditional positive regard, and congruent behaviors assist clients in building rapport and trust (Rogers, 1957). These same components are necessary in helping you and your classmates engage in trusting relationships and environments. Use your active listening skills and nonjudgmental actions with clients as well as your teachers, supervisors, and peers.

Power

Power: The ability to influence the behaviors of others through direct or indirect maneuvers.

Another often unspoken ability that is needed is that of personal and professional power. One definition of *power* is the ability to influence others due to the nature of the situation. There are many different layers of power in the helping professions. There is a power differential between counselor and client, counselor and supervisor, counselor/student and professor, and even intern and an existing counseling site. Each layer has its unique feature. In the varying combinations, one member of the dyad comes to the other member of the party because of expertise and skills that the other does not yet possess. Seeking guidance, wisdom, and knowledge from another automatically places you in a position with less power. Knowledge is power, and this power needs to be used cautiously and carefully.

In the counseling relationship, the counselor has the power from the beginning because the client is in a vulnerable state and is seeking help and relief. It is your job as a helping professional to lessen and/or eradicate that power through listening nonjudgmentally and allowing the client to solve individual concerns and make personal decisions.

Supervision: A structured approach to assist differing developmental and competency levels of helping professionals with a more experienced professional.

There is a parallel process with counseling and supervision. You enter into the supervisory relationship seeking guidance and wisdom. One large difference, though, is the fact that your supervisor and instructor, unlike counselor and client, do have an evaluative aspect to their job responsibilities. Because of evaluation and grading duties, faculty do have some power over your behaviors and attitudes as a student. In the beginning try to understand that all these relationships are new. Everyone has insecurities. Proceed slowly yet respectfully.

Sometimes you may be placed in a counseling setting that has a particular way of doing things, such as maintaining case notes and reports. As an enthusiastic and bright intern you may have exciting and more efficient ways of handling the system. You may see immediate changes that could solve a concern. Be sure to approach changing the agency cautiously and respectfully. You may need to listen and first seek a better understanding of the agency's history. You may need to keep personal opinions, reactions, and even great ideas to yourself until more bridges have been built and rapport has been created. In a later chapter you will learn that rapport with clients must be developed before you begin to confront them about necessary changes. This holds true for agency changes as well!

We all use power every day, and power can have both healthy and negative consequences. There are certain power skills you can utilize as a student to level out the playing field. As a student and counselor in training, the most important power skill you must utilize is to ask for what you need and clarify concerns. If you have the courage to do so, odds are you

Practical Reflection 4: Power Differentials

Describe a time when a helping professional used power inappropriately. What action could you have taken to display appropriate use of self-respect and clarification of personal needs?

_____

_____

_____

_____

will get what you desire. This works especially well if you believe your supervisor is using her or his power unfairly.

All the abilities discussed in this chapter are interwoven. Developing and using these abilities may be risky, but for the outcome of your field experience, it will be more risky not to use these abilities. All of the abilities described in this chapter are so essential for your field experience to be successful, for your supervisory relationship to prosper and grow, and for you to develop and refine your counseling skills.

Multicultural Issues

Another essential ability is the understanding of multicultural issues. The term *multiculturalism* has become increasingly inclusive over the years. Where once it referred specifically to ethnic or racial differences, multiculturalism now encompasses language, race and ethnicity, spiritual orientation, gender, sexual orientation, and many other factors. Cultural issues have become so broad that many now state that all counseling is multicultural and list the following factors as potential important components in the individual or group sessions (Ivey, Pedersen, & Ivey, 2001, 2–3):

- Family context
- Social systems context
- Demographic context
- Status context
- Life experience context

Practical Reflection 5: Multicultural Concerns

When have you been judgmental of another culture? Discuss the
many dimensions of that experience.

_____

_____

_____

_____

Culture is made up of all these issues and more. You and each of your
clients bring unique cultural experiences to the session. If your client is
going through a divorce and you have never had that experience, you are
engaged in a cross-cultural encounter even though you and your client
may be similar in many other ways. There is a culture of cancer survivors,
a culture of Persian Gulf veterans, and a culture of those who have immi-
grated to another country.

Field experience will test your ability to understand and be empathic.
There are those who say, "If you haven't been there, you can't understand." There is no question that if you have not been addicted to cocaine,
you likely cannot fully understand the issues your client faces. At the same
time, your own difficult life experiences will be helpful and your empathic
understanding, listening, and demeanor will make an important difference
in the life of your client.

Understanding the process of change allows you to guide others
through the system with your own special and unique orientation to the
world, even if you have not gone through that particular problem. As you
become more deeply immersed in the field experience, continue to
sharpen your understanding and awareness of the infinite multicultural
issues underlying all helping.

Positive Resources and Personal Strengths

A final ability that will prove invaluable to you is learned optimism,
demonstrating respect for both yourself and your clients. In your beginning skills course you began to appreciate the importance of the positive
asset search (Ivey and Ivey 2003). Drawing out the client's strengths,

Practical Reflection 6: Emphasizing Your Personal Strengths

Write down your personal strengths. Which of these strengths assisted you through a major transition and a difficult change during another period in your life? How are you utilizing these same resources currently in your field experience?

_____

_____

_____

_____

especially during painful and discouraging times, allows your client to regain personal power and focus on the concerns with a sense of renewed strength. Your client can remember that life has been better and not so difficult. If your client survived and surpassed other trying times, then this experience can be surpassed as well.

As with your clients, you are entering a somewhat scary and vulnerable field experience. Use the positive asset search to reframe your own challenges in your internship. By now you are beginning to know and understand yourself well. What are your strengths? Remember back now to another time in your life, when you were challenged and feeling insecure. Look at those resources to see which ones can generalize to your situation now. Perhaps special friends or family got you through, or you noticed that regular exercise regulated your stressors. Some of you may find that spiritual resources guided you. No one resource is the answer. We believe it is true that you can find strengths in your weaknesses and weaknesses in your strengths. Your optimistic attitude will allow the entire field experience to blossom.

Other Key Issues for the Success of Your Field Experience, Practicum, and Internship

Appreciating this time in your professional journey is paramount to your success. Here are a few additional resources that will help your practicum and internship be successful.

Scheduling Appointments.   To enjoy weekly supervision, first schedule weekly appointments set at regular times. This assures you and your supervisor that your weekly obligations are important to you. Do not assume your supervisor will arrange these meetings. Supervisors are very busy with other duties; your supervision is just one extra responsibility. As you set your weekly supervision times, be sure to discuss the expectations of the days and times you will serve. University calendars often conflict with agency and school calendars. Clarifying dates and the length of your stay is essential and will eliminate friction later. We tell our students that once you sign your placement contract, you need to abide by your site's calendar.

Resistance: Conscious or unconscious action designed to protect a client or supervisee from uncomfortable material or situations.

Owning Defensiveness.   You must not allow your insecurities to get in the way of receiving feedback. Early on in one of your first supervision sessions, as your supervisor is offering suggestions, you may find yourself thinking, "I know what I like and I like what I know. Stop offering me other ideas to confuse me!" At that moment begin to recognize and own any personal defensiveness. It is critical that you try not to be defensive and instead be receptive to your supervisors and peers. When you feel yourself shutting down, getting hurt or angry about someone's comments, and being generally inflexible, try to respond with "Please tell me more so I can better understand the intention and reasoning behind this." It is not easy to do, but remember there are a multitude of methods for counseling others. The more flexibility you learn, the more you will enjoy counseling those who are different from you, and the more helpful you can be to diverse populations. This natural defense is an emerging method of resistance. Just as clients may be resisting the counseling process, you might find yourself resisting the supervision process. Being aware of this natural way of protection is a first step toward understanding yourself better.

Understanding the Complexities of the Change Process.   This next situation will eventually happen to you, as it has occurred with every person in the counseling profession and every person in the world. Sometimes you will just feel stuck in the counseling session. Theories and techniques do not work and you feel as if you don't comprehend any of the needed conceptual ideas for your client. Remember that change is a difficult journey. It is, however, one of the few constants in the world, so it is important that you understand about the change process, for you as well as your clients. Most of us do not like change. It goes against the status quo, and often our bad situation or techniques are just fine; at least they are familiar.

Carl Jung made a similar point in 1954. If something is not working, don't keep doing the same thing! If you follow his sage advice, whenever you feel stuck or confused, remember to experiment with another technique or theory. We think confusion is a healthy place to be. If you are confused, you are not stuck. You are moving to another place, the stagnation has left, and the change process has begun. A skilled plumber once said, "It's not the mistakes you make; it's the recovery skills that count!"

An example of the change process is illustrated in a story about a small boy named Sam. He lived with his very strict father and feared him very much. One day, Sam and his friends were playing baseball in the front yard, and Sam hit the ball into the neighbor's side window, shattering it into little pieces. The children scattered in all directions knowing they were all in big trouble. Sam tried to think what to do. He knew his father would be furious, because he had told the children not to play ball in the front yard. Sam could not force himself to tell his father the truth. His fear of his father's punishment was greater than the pain of telling the truth and facing the future consequences. Very few of us are willing to change, not our clients or ourselves, until the fear of the unknown is less than the current pain!

This story can be seen in the opposite light as well, by stating that you will not change unless the current pain is greater than the fear of the unknown. So anytime you begin to struggle in your field experience, sit down and face your pain and fears. Decide what you can do to move to the next phase. This would be a great topic for your individual supervision sessions!

Needing a Personal Counselor.   The topics of supervision will vary greatly. You have been encouraged to ask for what you want and pick the brains of your supervisors. Sometimes, though, you need to let the supervision process unfold naturally. Sometimes, you won't even know what it is you need or want. That, too, is all right. Sometimes you may need to talk about you and not the client. If you let that happen, your client will indirectly benefit, because you will have allowed yourself to deal with elements in your life that may be interfering with your role as a counselor. We are not suggesting that you engage in counseling with your supervisor. That is crossing an ethical boundary of dual relationships, but you can deal with immediate concerns. If there is more to the issue, please allow your supervisor to refer you to a helping professional or find a counselor for yourself. Every person can benefit from personal counseling. Your field experience is a very stressful time, so personal counseling would serve as a useful tool and resource.

Transference and Countertransference.   There is another way you can tell if you may need counseling during your practicum and internship. If you think your supervisor is "the best thing since sliced bread," "he

Transference: Passing personal characteristics of significant others in past relationships onto a therapist, supervisor, or others.

must be the best supervisor in the entire world," or "she doesn't understand anything about this case," you may be experiencing the phenomena of transference. This also shows when you think about your supervisor frequently.

Sometime during your field experience, you may be asked whether you like all your clients all the time. Many students new to the helping professions will hesitate and answer, "Yes!" It truly is healthy to like and even dislike clients. However, liking a client too much and disliking clients too much are particularly dangerous transferential issues. When this happens to you, and it will, be sure to discuss it with your supervisors.

Be cautious of extreme emotions during the supervisory process. This intense experience and often deep supervisory relationship is rich and fertile ground for personal growth and unfinished business with others. Your supervisor may be the one person who can help you to deal with old issues. If the wounds are deep, this is the perfect time to seek personal counseling in addition to supervision. From several decades of providing counseling services, it seemed as if every time we had unfinished business in our lives, it would walk right into our offices! It is then that we know it is time to enter into personal counseling.

Countertransference: A phenomenon where a person in authority transfers personal qualities of significant others from the past onto subordinates.

Don't be afraid to seek counseling when you need it the most. The flip side of this coin is, of course, countertransference. You may find sometimes that your supervisor has issues too. That should be of no surprise to you; everyone does. If you feel that your supervisor is placing unfair expectations on you or placing emotions onto you that are not yours, please have the courage to address that with him or her. Often it will be the immediacy you need to assist you both in growing. If this doesn't work, contact your university supervisor.

Practical Reflection 7: Analyzing Past Transference and Countertransference Issues

Discuss with your classmates any times you now realize may have been transference or countertransference issues.

_____

_____

_____

_____

Summary and Personal Integration

This chapter emphasizes the importance of getting started correctly by identifying fears and concerns that may get in your way. Issues that were presented were:

- courage
- risk taking
- goal setting
- feedback
- respect
- power
- multicultural issues
- resources

Individual strengths were identified; each of you come to your field experience with unique skills and expertise. Try not to compare your strengths with those of others but focus on your current strengths and resources. Take a deep breath—you are just getting started, remember?

Practical Reflection 8: Integration

What Chapter 1 constructs will be the most helpful to you as you begin your field experience?

_____

_____

_____

_____

References

Bailey, A. (1986). Faculty leaders in profile. *Change* 18, July/August: 24–32, 37–47.
Curtis, R. C. (2000). Using goal-setting strategies to enrich the practicum and internship experiences of beginning counselors. *Journal of Humanistic Counseling, Education and Development* 38:194–205.

Ivey, A. E., and Ivey, M. B. (2003). *Intentional Interviewing and Counseling*, 5th ed. Pacific Grove, Calif.: Brooks/Cole.

Ivey, A., Pedersen, P., and Ivey, M. (2001). *Intentional Group Counseling*. Pacific Grove, Calif.: Brooks/Cole.

Jung, C. G. (1954). *The Practice of Psychotherapy*, vol. 16. London: Routledge & Kegan Paul.

Rogers, C. 1957. The necessary and sufficient conditions of therapeutic personality change. *Journal of Consulting Psychology* 21:95–103.

LISTENING TO TAPES AND ANALYZING CASES: MICROCOUNSELING SUPERVISION

⇨ *If you take what your client gives you, you will rarely be lost in the counseling process. If you do get lost, attend, attend, and attend!*

OVERVIEW

GOALS

KEY CONCEPTS: MICROCOUNSELING SUPERVISION

THE THREE COMPONENTS OF MICROCOUNSELING SUPERVISION

REVIEWING MICROCOUNSELING SKILLS WITH INTENTION

PRACTICAL REFLECTION 1: REVIEWING SKILLS WITH INTENTION

CLASSIFYING SKILLS WITH MASTERY

PRACTICAL REFLECTION 2: CLASSIFYING SKILLS WITH MASTERY

PROCESSING SUPERVISORY NEEDS

SUPERVISORY PROCESS

PRACTICAL REFLECTION 3: SUMMARIZING AND PROCESSING SKILLS

USES OF THE CIRF

CASE PRESENTATION

PRACTICAL REFLECTION AND SELF-ASSESSMENT 4: ESTABLISHING YOUR COUNSELING SKILLS BASELINE

PRACTICAL REFLECTION 5: UNDERSTANDING MICROCOUNSELING SUPERVISION

SUMMARY AND PERSONAL INTEGRATION

PRACTICAL REFLECTION 6: INTEGRATION

REFERENCES

RESOURCES A THROUGH E

OVERVIEW

Listening to interview tapes and analyzing case presentations are essential teaching strategies for every helping profession educational program. This chapter reviews basic interviewing skills that are used in some fashion in every theoretical orientation and counseling interview. The chapter focuses on the Microcounseling Supervision Model (MSM) providing a vocabulary guide and a framework for constant examination of your personal counseling style.

The Counseling Interview Rating Form (CIRF), an integral part of the MSM, is an instrument that can be utilized for qualitative and quantitative feedback for counseling interviews. You will examine and practice your interviewing skills using the CIRF. Other methods of supervision will be presented later in the text, but Microcounseling Supervision is presented first as a foundation for listening to counseling interviews and reviewing necessary skills.

GOALS

1. Label and identify which counseling skills are being used during one of your videotaped counseling interviews using the Counseling Interview Rating Form (CIRF).
2. Use the CIRF to quantify and qualify other students' videotapes.
3. Deliver constructive feedback to others and appreciate the importance of individual constructive feedback.
4. Identify the three basic components of the Microcounseling Supervision Model (MSM).
5. Plan and deliver a concise case presentation.

KEY CONCEPTS: MICROCOUNSELING SUPERVISION

Two of the most important learning strategies in your field experience are listening to counseling tapes and analyzing case presentations. Obtaining feedback from your classroom supervisor, on-site supervisor, and your supervisory peers about your video- or audiotapes and case presentations is crucial to your personal development and growth as a new counselor and helping professional. This feedback is essential to you and your clients' growth. In this chapter, a method for providing personal feedback is presented using the Microcounseling Supervision Model (MSM) and the corresponding Counseling Interview Rating Form (CIRF).

Microcounseling Supervision: A supervision model that allows you to work independently and/or in peer group supervision to understand the basic fundamentals of the counseling process and interview. Microcounseling skills are used in almost every model of supervision, and this model of supervision builds a strong foundation for needed basic skills. It has three stages: (1) Reviewing Skills with Intention, (2) Classifying Skills with Mastery, and (3) Understanding the Supervisory Process.

Counseling Interview Rating Form (CIRF): The Counseling Interview Rating Form is an instrument that provides a method for evaluating the five stages of the counseling interview and microcounseling and influencing skills. A quantitative score can be derived as well as qualitative comments. A copy of the CIRF is included at the end of this chapter; you may also use a supplemental CD-ROM and click on the instrument icon to print additional copies of the CIRF.

The Microcounseling Supervision Model (MSM) is a standardized approach assisting you in reviewing, offering feedback, teaching, and evaluating microcounseling skills. There are three major components to the MSM: (1) reviewing skills with intention, (2) classifying skills with mastery, and (3) processing supervisory needs. Its tenets are based on microcounseling skills first reported by Ivey, Normington, Miller, Morrill, and Haase (1968), and all the skills correspond to the five stages of the counseling interview.

Microcounseling Supervision offers a way for you to learn to give constructive feedback that incorporates your strengths and areas for improvements by following the format of the CIRF. In beginning skills classes you were encouraged to give others feedback. Usually the comments were very positive, "You were great," or "I liked the way you paraphrased." During your field experiences, though, more than positive feedback must be given. If constructive feedback is not provided to each of you as students in field experiences, progress will be stagnant and perhaps nonexistent.

We discussed in Chapter 1 that feedback is not about you personally, but it is about a particular skill or process. Also remember that it is your responsibility to ask your peer group, supervisor, and instructor for specific needs and wants during your supervisory time together. Feedback that is requested is best received. Request what you want and need. You know where you struggle, even if you don't know exactly what to ask. When you take ownership for your counseling progress, you will feel less insecure and vulnerable about your counseling style, supervision, and having others view your counseling videotapes!

As you may remember, microcounseling skills are used in some fashion in every theoretical orientation. You practiced these skills in your beginning skills courses and in every course thereafter. Many of you role-played using these same microcounseling skills. Therefore, the beauty of Microcounseling Supervision is that it teaches you, the student, and your supervisors a natural method for reviewing your counseling tapes and offering feedback, regardless of theoretical orientation.

Lambert and Ogles (1997) described microcounseling skills as an approach that facilitates the general purposes of psychotherapy no matter what the theoretical orientation. The effectiveness of microcounseling skills training has been researched for decades (Miller, Morril, & Uhlemann, 1970; Scissons, 1993). In 1989, Baker and Daniels analyzed 81 studies on microcounseling skills training. They concluded that microcounseling skills training surpassed both the no training and attention-placebo-control comparison. Daniels (2003) has followed microcounseling research for many years and now has identified over 450 data-based studies on the model.

Russell-Chapin and Sherman (2000) found, even with the effectiveness of the microcounseling approach, little consistency in the strategies used to actually measure and evaluate counseling students' skills and videotapes: "The need for quantifying counselor skills becomes increasingly important as the counseling profession continues to develop and refine standards for counselor competence" (p. 116). The CIRF was designed in response to the need to accurately and effectively supervise students' counseling videotapes and live supervision sessions (Russell-Chapin & Sherman, 2000). The CIRF has a variety of functions, but it is mostly used as a method of providing positive and corrective feedback for your student counseling tapes. Refer to a blank CIRF (Resource C) at the end of this chapter and follow along to learn how to use this form. You may also choose to view the supplemental video to observe students using this form during an actual live Microcounseling Supervision session or use the CD-ROM demonstrating each of the microcounseling skills.

THE THREE COMPONENTS OF MICROCOUNSELING SUPERVISION

Reviewing Microcounseling Skills With Intention

The first component of the MSM is essential to the efficacy and efficiency of the remaining sections. Once you are comfortable and secure with defining and reviewing the microcounseling skills, then you can rapidly enter into the second phase. However, please initially take the time to ensure that you understand each individual skill definition along with the underlying intention of that skill. *Intention* is choosing the best potential response from among the many possible options.

Skill Definitions and Glossary: Forty-three counseling skills are used in the CIRF. Skill definition can be located in two manners. All skills are defined in Resource A. Each skill is also defined and demonstrated in a supplemental microcounseling CD-ROM. On the CD-ROM, view the demonstrated skills by clicking on the skill you want to review. Each skill has a definition, an actual demonstration of that skill, a counselor script, and one additional example of that skill.

Practical Reflection 1: Reviewing Skills With Intention

A glossary of the microcounseling skills with their intentionality is provided in Resource A at the end of this chapter. Read through the list of skills by yourself and circle the skills you do not understand or the ones that do not seem familiar. List the skills that are unfamiliar to you. Begin to talk among your classmates about the unfamiliar skills and their intentionality. Once your review is complete, you can move to the second stage of Microcounseling Supervision.

_____

_____

_____

_____

Intentionality: Selecting specific counseling skills in anticipation of particular interviewing results.

You are not looking for the "right" solution and skill, but you are selecting responses to adapt your counseling style to meet the differing needs and culture of clients (Ivey & Ivey, 2003). With intentionality you anticipate specific interviewing results if you use certain skills! For example, if you want your client to continue expressing emotions, a basic reflection of feeling would be a wise skill to choose. Your client laments, "Today was my little boy's first day of kindergarten!" The counselor's reflection of feeling is, "There must be many differing emotions going on inside. You could be sad, lonely, scared yet excited!" Let's get started in the first step of Microcounseling Supervision by practicing, defining, and reviewing all the microcounseling skills.

Classifying Skills With Mastery

One of the easiest methods to begin the second stage of classifying skills with mastery is to have examples of someone else demonstrating the microcounseling skills and their uses. Do you remember the case of Rachel from the Preface? She was introduced as the older client Lori faced her first counseling interview. An edited transcript of that session follows. As you read the transcript from the session, classify the microskills that Lori used in the space provided.

We will classify the first response with you. Lori is just listening and nodding. You would classify that skill as a "minimal encourager." Was

Lori's skill done with intention? In other words, was Lori successful with her choice of skills? In this case, we think Lori's choice did work, because Rachel continues talking and her resistance begins to lessen. Continue classifying Lori's counseling responses. Then compare your ideas with our classifications on the following page.

As you read and classify the skills in this session, note that Lori's life experience is indeed different from Rachel's. The two people have varying cultural experiences. Acknowledging that difference early in the interview is important. If you are a white European-American and your client is African-American, for example, the same frank discussion of differences can be helpful. Similarly, if you work with a gay adolescent and you are heterosexual or a younger counselor working with an older client, upfront discussion of the differences can be important in developing trust. But always do this with sensitivity and careful client observation. There are no hard and fast rules on this important issue, but generally it is considered best to explore differences.

Practical Reflection 2: Classifying Skills With Mastery

Example Interview: The Case of Rachel

The following is a transcript of Lori's first counseling session. Rachel, the client, was hesitant to join into the counseling relationship. Rachel immediately took control of the session. She chose not to sit down and wandered around the counseling office.

Notice in this example that the Microskill Classification column is on the left and the transcript is on the right-hand side of the page. Classify each of Lori's counseling responses. Then turn to Resource B to compare your classifications with ours.

MICROSKILL CLASSIFICATION	TRANSCRIPT OF RACHEL AND LORI
	1. RACHEL: *Honey, what could you possibly have to offer? You are a child with very little life experience, and you will never be able to help or understand my problems.*
Minimal encourager	2. LORI: *(nods and listens)*
	3. RACHEL: *How could you ever help me?*
	4. LORI: *Rachel, you are probably correct. I have not lived as long as you, and I don't have as much life experience*

as you. All I can do is listen to you and see if a counseling relationship develops. How does that sound to you?

5. RACHEL: *(finally sits down) It sounds fine, but it won't do any good. You see John and I were happily married for 50 years! He died quite suddenly 6 months ago, and I just don't know what to do.*

6. LORI: *Having your husband be an important part of your life for so long and die unexpectedly must be devastating. I am very sorry.*

7. RACHEL: *(pausing and looking at Lori) Do you have any idea what this is like?*

8. LORI: *I truly don't know what it is like to lose a husband, but I do know what is it like to lose a loved one; my father died when I was 25. I was scared and very sad.*

9. RACHEL: *You are right, it is not the same, but at least you know some of what it feels like.*

10. LORI: *So we have a few things in common, and one of your concerns we could work on in counseling is about the loss of your husband. Is that right?*

11. RACHEL: *Yes, I would like to work on that, and I guess, I'd like to talk about what to do with myself now that John is gone. We did so much together; it is like my left arm has been cut off.*

12. LORI: *Having John gone hits you at many different levels. Not only was he your companion with whom you did everything, it is also like a piece of you is missing as well.*

13. RACHEL: *Yes, yes. There are many different levels. All three of our children are grown, but they so miss their dad and now they are calling me constantly to see if I am all right. Honestly, they are driving me crazy with their questions and concern! My youngest wants me to leave our home and move away with him.*

14. LORI: *Rachel, I noticed that when you began talking of your children, your voice became higher and louder; you almost seemed agitated. Tell me more about your children and your relationship.*

15. RACHEL: *I love my children, but we all have our own lives. It feels like now they suddenly think I am incapable of living by myself. I am only 71 years old! I still drive my car; I play duplicate bridge; I tutor first*

Practical Reflection 2: Classifying Skills With Mastery (continued)

graders in reading . . . well, I mean I used to do those things.

16. LORI: *Let me see if I am truly understanding the situation. You miss your husband very much and are lonely, but recently your three children are trying to coddle you and even persuade you to possibly move away and live with them. You believe you are quite capable of living on your own without John, as you used to do many independent things. Many activities you and John did together, but some of these things sound as if you even did them without John. Am I correctly understanding the gist of it all?*

17. RACHEL: *Yes, yes. (Rachel became silent again; Lori sat quietly with her for several very long minutes.) I miss the things John and I used to do! I miss my old life.*

18. LORI: *Rachel, what do you miss about your old life?*

19. RACHEL: *We were both retired, so we had the freedom to travel. We went everywhere. I have so many memories of our travels and years together. We have many friends in this town and throughout the country.*

20. LORI: *Those memories serve as a reminder of the great times together but they also remind you of your losses. Rachel, how many of those friends have you contacted recently?*

21. RACHEL: *I received hundreds of cards and memorials. I answered each one with a hand-written thank-you note. But, I have not contacted anyone for a get-together since John's death.*

22. LORI: *Your loneliness goes deeper than John. Am I close?*

23. RACHEL: *(crying) I miss my entire old life.*

24. LORI: *The sadness and loss seem overwhelming.*

25. RACHEL: *I don't know what to do.*

26. LORI: *Rachel, you have gone through 6 very difficult months. Even in this office you have exhibited many varying emotions, from shock to sadness to anger. These are very similar to the stages of grief. Your feelings are very normal and valid. The consequences of John's death seem to have shattered your old life. Let's set up several*

counseling goals to help you restructure your life and feelings.

27. RACHEL: *I wouldn't even know what goals to set.*
28. LORI: *You have already offered me several ideas, and there are many alternative ways to start. The first goal is to openly share your grief with others. You have done a wonderful job in here just by telling me your varying feelings and thoughts. I would like you to be this specific with your three children as well. Between now and our next session, would you be willing to contact each of your children, telling them how you miss John and their dad and also how you feel about their coddling?*

29. RACHEL: *Yes, I will call each child.*
30. LORI: *The only other goal I would like us to set today is that you will contact one of your duplicate bridge friends to find out the next arranged game time. Are you willing to do that?*

31. RACHEL: *(smiles slowly) I am not sure about that one, but I will try.*
32. LORI: *We have about 15 minutes left in our session. We have covered a lot of territory in our short time. I think I understand the depth of your loss. John must have been a great partner. You miss him so much, and you are lonely. You would like to have your old life back. Topping it all off are your children who love you very much and are very concerned about you living alone. I have also learned you have given up much of what you used to enjoy such as bridge, tutoring, and traveling.*

33. RACHEL: *We did cover a lot of territory. Until we started talking, I didn't realize how much I have lost.*
34. LORI: *What part of the counseling session helps you understand why you have been so sad?*

35. RACHEL: *Lots of things help me understand, but I am still somewhat confused.*
36. LORI: *Rachel, let's clarify even more then. What did we work on today that makes sense to you?*

37. RACHEL: *Well, what I said earlier about not just John's dying, but I am sad about losing so much of my previous life.*
38. LORI: *You are sad about many of your losses, and today you stated that you are willing to regain control of at*

Practical Reflection 2: Classifying Skills With Mastery (continued)

	least two areas in your life. You will let your children know you love them but are very capable of living alone and you said you would call a duplicate bridge friend.
	39. RACHEL: *I did say that, didn't I?!*
	40. LORI: *Yes, you did! I took from today's session that your feelings and grief are, indeed, valid and very normal. Rachel, you came here today very hesitant, and when you saw me, you knew I couldn't be of help. How are you feeling about us now?*
	41. RACHEL: *I still think you are very young. But you said you would listen and you did. Thank you, my dear child.*
	42. LORI: *Rachel, it was a pleasure to work with you. What would you like to do about setting up another appointment?*

Now that you have had a chance to review and classify many of the essential skills, you may recognize that several skills are closely correlated and could be identified in several categories. For example, take a look at Lori's number 20 response. Lori stated, "Those memories serve as a reminder of the great times together, but they also remind you of your losses." We classified that response as a reflection of meaning because the purpose was to expand Rachel's own thoughts. It could also be an example of exploration/understanding of the concern.

Talk to your classmates about those similarities, differences, and whether the skill produced anticipated results. You are using the basic skills intentionally when you think ahead to what might happen as a result of skill usage. If that anticipated result does not occur, you can change your use of skills to facilitate client growth. The more you can articulate those differences and similarities, the sooner you will be able to choose which skills may be more intentionally needed at which times!

Processing Supervisory Needs

Now it is time for you to enter the third component of the MSM and begin summarizing and processing these skills on the CIRF (Resource C) as well as other important dimensions of the session. Before you begin the actual using of the CIRF, you need additional information about the instrument itself.

The Counseling Interview Rating Form   A major component of Microcounseling Supervision is the CIRF. The CIRF was originally developed for a counselor education program, but it has been used in both educational and clinical settings. The CIRF is the structured underpinning of Microcounseling Supervision; it provides a format for evaluating the five stages of the counseling interview as described by Ivey and Ivey (2003) and the microcounseling skills used in the counseling interview.

The CIRF was created by including the essential listening and influencing skills taught in many helping professional programs. Two categories of skills are included: (1) listening and influencing skills (Ivey et al. 1968) and (2) counseling interview stages (Ivey 1994). The CIRF is divided into six sections that correspond to the five stages of a counseling interview, plus one additional section on professionalism. The vocabulary used for the five stages of the interview are: (1) Opening, (2) Exploration, (3) Action, (4) Problem Solving, and (5) Closing sections. Listed within each section are skills or tasks that are seen in that stage of the interview. The Opening section, for example, includes the specific criteria of greeting, role definition, administrative tasks, and beginning.

Scoring the CIRF   While watching one of your current videotapes or participating in a live counseling supervision session, you will complete the CIRF and tally the number of times a certain skill is used with frequency marks. If you saw the skill demonstrated five different times, you would mark a frequency tally each time. Values are assigned after the counseling session to indicate the level of mastery achieved for each skill. Write in the ratings of 1, 2, or 3 for each of the 43 listed skills that were observed.

Ivey and Ivey (2003) describe *mastery* as using the skills with intention with an observable, desired effect on the client. You would offer a score of 1 if you only saw a counselor using that skill with little or no effect on the client. A score of 2 says the counselor used the skill with mastery and intention and a score of 3 says the counselor was demonstrating and teaching a new skill or concept to the client. As you can imagine, a score of 3 is used sparingly.

The CIRF includes space for comments next to each skill, so any reviewer can make notes or write the counselor's actual statements while viewing the tape. These comments are extremely important to the supervisory session, because they offer the counselor true examples of skills and processes used during the interview. The last page of the CIRF consists of space for providing written feedback on the strengths and areas for improvements. During Microcounseling Supervision, all peer supervisors and the instructor will use the narrative space to provide constructive feedback.

If using the CIRF for quantifying counseling sessions into grades, the total values are tallied, with an A corresponding to 52 points and higher (i.e., at least 90 percent of the total points). This cut-off score requires scoring in the mastery range on all the essential skills denoted by an X on the CIRF. Essential skills are those deemed necessary for an effective interview as determined by the CIRF authors and the microcounseling approach to training (Russell-Chapin & Sherman, 2000).

SUPERVISORY PROCESS

Practical Reflection 3: Summarizing and Processing Skills

Now turn to the CIRF (Resource C). Again use the interview with Lori and the Case of Rachel and begin summarizing skill usage with frequency tallies. Go through the transcript again and use a frequency tally for each of Lori's counseling responses. At the end of the session or during each response, see which of Lori's responses represent basic mastery and active mastery. Remember, *basic mastery* is being able to demonstrate the skill during the interview; *active mastery* shows Lori producing specific and intentional results from the chosen counseling skill.

The final step is to compare your ratings with ours (Resource D). In a regular classroom, this final step will be discussing your ratings with your classmates and instructor. Once the CIRF has been tallied by the members of the supervisory team, the narrative process for Microcounseling

Supervision can begin. If you are the student counselor presenting the video and case presentation, you have been asked to prepare needed supervisory questions and concerns. These issues are addressed as a team in a round-robin fashion going over supervisory concerns, strengths, and areas for improvement. The very last question asked of you will be, "What did you learn in supervision today that will assist you in more effectively working with this client?"

Many of these comments may come from the Strengths and Area for Improvement area of the CIRF. The comments on these sections will help you immensely to progress forward. Lori's comments were from her supervisor, Dr. Ivey. After reading the next section on Case Presentations, you will discover that many of Lori's supervisory questions and concerns were answered.

USES OF THE CIRF

The CIRF is useful as an evaluative tool for supervisors and peers and for self-evaluation. By using this form as a central foundation to Microcounseling Supervision, you can approach supervision time with less vulnerability; the environment to supervision is not threatening but validating. In addition to being an evaluation tool, the CIRF is an excellent teaching tool. Use the CIRF to identify areas and skills frequently used and those skills not being demonstrated effectively.

Case Presentation

Another essential skills for any helping professional is creating a clear case presentation. This is an important part of Microcounseling Supervision because the structure allows you to orally present your confidential, written case study to a small group of your counseling peers and instructor.

You have already received permission from your client and have placed that Consent Form in the client's file. Then you preview your videotape and begin writing down major components of the case. Here is one method in written outline and narrative form to assist you in professionally sharing essential information about your client. Your case presentation can be offered first to your supervision group, and then the videotape is watched in conjunction with scoring the CIRF, or you may prefer to view the counseling tape first and then present the case presentation. Either approach is fine, but make a strategic decision about the order. We sometimes prefer to watch the videotape first and score the CIRF; the case presentation may skew some classmates' opinions about certain client characteristics and situations. Either way you will need to share your supervisory questions and concerns.

Decide in what order to make the case presentation, and be sure to watch the videotape from beginning to end. It is often better to begin the supervisory processing by having your classmates voice your strengths. Then request the feedback you need. As trust continues to build, your classmates may offer insights that you have not seen. An easy method for offering feedback is to follow the CIRF format. Ask your colleagues to actually state the comments you demonstrated showing particular strengths and even liabilities.

Providing written copies of the report at the very beginning of the case presentation works well. It seems helpful to all to have the information in front of each team or class member. After the supervision session is over, all copies go back to the supervisee to destroy. Even though client names have been shortened, blanked out, or used in initial form, it is wise to shred these reports for confidentiality reasons.

You may want to collect all the CIRFs to see all the comments from your peers and supervisor. At this point, add all your scores and average the tape score for a final tape grade. You will notice on the CIRF that Lori received a score for her interview with Rachel. She received a total of 58 points out of a possible 86 points, if each skill were demonstrated with active mastery. How does that compare with your scoring of the Case of Rachel?

Practical Reflection and Self-Assessment 4: Establishing Your Counseling Skills Baseline

Now that you are familiar with the CIRF, watch one of your previous counseling videotapes that is relatively recent. Your self-assessment task is to classify each of the microcounseling skills you demonstrated. Using another blank (Resource E) CIRF, place a frequency tally in the column marked Frequency every time you demonstrate a skill.

Be sure to write down as much of the actual statements in the column labeled Comments. Once your entire tape is classified, go back and offer the ratings in the column marked Skill Mastery Rating. You can add up your scores if you want, but right now the grade is not the most important consideration. This initial baseline of skills helps you identify those skills you are using often and with intention. Also look for those counseling skills that you avoid and are not being used. The skills you are not choosing to use are just as telling as your frequently identified skills! Use this baseline information to assist you in goal setting and future practice.

Practical Reflection 5: Understanding Microcounseling Supervision

As you practice using the Microcounseling Supervision Model, which of the three components will be most helpful to you now: Reviewing Skills with Intention, Classifying Skills with Mastery or Understanding the Supervisory Process?

_____

_____

_____

_____

SUMMARY AND PERSONAL INTEGRATION

Listening to interview tapes and analyzing case presentations are essential to the growth of novice helping professionals. To help facilitate those skills, the following points were presented in Chapter 2:

- The Microcounseling Supervision Model (MSM) can be used to assist you in building a foundation necessary for effective counseling and developmental growth. It provides natural building blocks for better understanding basic attending behaviors and influencing skills.
- The Counseling Interview Rating Form (CIRF) assists you in developing a system for reciprocal supervision where you, your colleagues, and your instructor can offer constructive feedback. This begins a magic dance of supervision where an easy and natural flow can encourage you to be receptive to new ideas and interventions. The CIRF not only reviews and teaches you how to classify specific skills and behaviors but how to evaluate their intention as well. Finally, the CIRF assists you in examining whether the goals of each interview stage are being achieved. Practice using the CIRF and experience the natural flow of Microcounseling Supervision.

Practical Reflection 6: Integration

Based on the information gained in Chapter 2, list at least three skills and/or strategies that will assist you in more effectively listening to client tapes and analyzing cases.

_____

_____

_____

_____

REFERENCES

Baker, S. B., and Daniels, T. (1989). Integrating research on the microcounseling program: A meta-analysis. *Journal of Counseling Psychology* 36:213–22.

Daniels, T. (2003). Microcounseling research: What over 450 data-based studies reveal. In *Leader Guide to Intentional Interviewing and Counseling*, edited by A. Ivey, M. Ivey, and R. Marx. Pacific Grove, Calif.: Brooks/Cole.

Ivey, A. E. & Ivey, M. B. (2003). *Intentional Interviewing and Counseling*, 5th ed. Pacific Grove, Calif.: Brooks/Cole.

Ivey, A. E., Miller, C., Morrill, W., and Haase, R. (1968). Microcounseling and attending behavior: An approach to prepracticum counselor training. *Journal of Counseling Psychology* 15, no. 5:1–12.

Lambert, M. J., and Ogles, B. M. (1997). The effectiveness of psychotherapy supervision. In *The Handbook of Psychotherapy Supervision* (pp 421–46). Edited by C. E. Watkins, Jr. New York: Wiley.

Miller, C., Morrill, W., and Uhlemann, M. (1970). An experimental study of pre-practicum training in communicating test results. *Counselor Education and Supervision* 9:171–7.

Russell-Chapin, L. A., and Sherman, N. E. (2000). The counseling interview rating form: A teaching and evaluation tool for counselor education. *British Journal of Guidance and Counseling* 28, no. 1:115–24.

Scissons, E. H. (1993). *Counseling for Results: Principles and Practices of Helping Professions*. Pacific Grove, Calif.: Brooks/Cole.

RESOURCE A: GLOSSARY OF CIRF SKILLS

Opening/Developing Rapport Skills

SKILL AND DEFINITION	INTENTION
Greeting: A simple acknowledgment to the client.	Build rapport.
Role definition/expectation: Description of the counselor roles and intention of counseling; confidentiality and its limit.	Provide structure.
Administrative tasks: Procedures necessary for counseling such as Client Rights, Payment, Scheduling and Intake Forms.	Clarify procedures.
Beginning: An open-ended question demonstrating to the client the interview is starting, such as "What do you want to work on today?"	Offer an expansive method of beginning the interview.

Exploration Phase/Defining the Problem Microskills

SKILL AND DEFINITION	INTENTION
Empathy/rapport: Behaviors and attitudes indicating understanding and active listening.	Encourage the client to continue.
Respect: Offering genuine acknowledgment of client's concerns.	Build rapport.
Nonverbal matching: Using body gestures and positions to mirror the client's.	Build rapport and acceptance.
Minimal encourager: An occasional word, nod, or "uh, huh," encouraging the client to continue.	Encourage the client to continue.
Paraphrasing: Actively rephrasing in the counselor's own words and perceptions what the client has stated, such as "Your mother died recently and you miss her."	Create understanding of client's words.

(continued)

RESOURCE A CONTINUED

Pacing/leading: Allowing the client to direct the interview flow by counselor matching of words and verbal intonation; counselor directing when interview flow needs transition.

Encourages comfort, discourages resistance.

Verbal tracking: Consistent following of client's verbal direction and themes.

Create continuity from client's content.

Reflect feeling: Paraphrase the client's feelings, such as "How sad that must be."

Increases understanding of client's feelings.

Reflect meaning: Paraphrasing the client's deeper level of experience, such as "Death can be an ending and perhaps a beginning."

Increases wider perspective.

Clarifications: Eliminating confusion of terms by seeking clearer understanding of client's words.

Eliminates confusion of terms.

Open-ended questions: Asking global questions for the purpose of receiving maximum or infinite amount of information such as "What do you miss the most about your mother?"

Receives maximum or infinite amount of information.

Summarization: Paraphrasing a cluster of themes or topics during the interview, providing transition and/or closure.

Provides for transition and/or closure.

Behavioral description: Informing the client of what you observe of a behavior or mannerism: "When we began talking about sister and mother's relationship, I noticed your eyes teared up and you moved your chair away from me."

Eliminates assumptions about behaviors and assists in client awareness.

Appropriate closed questions: An intentional question used to obtain a finite amount of information, such as "How old were you when your mother died?"

Gains finite amounts of information.

Perception check: A periodic moment to ask the client if your perceptions or ideas about the concern are accurate: "Is that accurate concerning your sister and mother's relationship?"

Check counselor's perception and accuracy.

Silence: Allowing purposeful, quiet reflection during the interview.

Allows for purposeful, quiet reflection during the interview.

Focusing: Consistent and intentional selection of topic, construct, and/or direction in the session.

Aids in direction of the session.

Feedback: Offering information to the client concerning attitude and behavior, such as "Last week you came here with crumpled clothes, but today you have washed your hair and clothes."

Provides awareness about behaviors, thoughts, and feelings.

Problem-Solving Skills/Defining Skills

SKILL AND DEFINITION

INTENTION

Definition of goals: Statements stipulating directions, outcomes, and goals for the client.

Stipulates directions for counseling.

Exploration/understanding of concerns: Using needed microskills to discover the nature of the concern.

Collects essential information about client's concern.

Development/evaluation of alternatives: Assisting the client in creating a myriad of options for problem solution; assessing the potential and possibilities surrounding each option.

Assesses the potential and possibilities surrounding each option.

Implement alternative: Actively planning and articulating necessary steps for placing option into reality.

Assists in putting ideas into action.

Special techniques: Any counseling intervention used to assist the client in deeper understanding of the concern, such as imagery or an Empty Chair.

Provides for the needs of individual clients.

Process counseling: Helping the client to understand special themes and dynamics involved in the problem, such as loss and fear.

Allows for deeper understanding of client issues.

(*continued*)

RESOURCE A CONTINUED

Action Phase/Confronting Incongruities

SKILL AND DEFINITION	INTENTION
Immediacy: Stopping the interview and immediately seeking clarification about a dynamic or observation in the client or between the counselor and client: "You stopped talking after your dad was mentioned. What is happening right now?"	Keeps the sessions in the here and now.
Self-disclosure: Offering relevant, helpful and appropriate information about the counselor for the purpose of client assistance: "When my father died, I was 21 years old. My compass was gone, and I was lost."	Assists the client in universality of life.
Confrontation: Pointing out client discrepancies between words, behaviors, and thoughts.	Helps the client to become aware of thoughts and actions.
Directives: An influencing statement specifying an action or thought for the client to take: "The next time you visit your Mother's grave, I suggest you write a poem expressing your fears and loneliness."	Offers needed structure for differing developmental client needs; shows acceptance.
Logical consequences: Exploring the results/consequences of the client's actions and solutions; the consequences can be natural or logical.	Points out results of client decisions.
Interpretation: Presenting a new frame of reference on the client's concern, possibly through different theoretical orientations: "It may be that the death of your mother forces you to be alone with yourself and your own fears."	Presents a new frame of reference on the client's concern.

Closing/Generalization

SKILL AND DEFINITION	INTENTION
Summarization of content/feeling: Closing the session by tying together themes involving subject matter and emotions.	Ties together the counseling themes.
Review of plan: Organizing the desired outcome into a plan and reviewing it with the client.	Reminds the client of previously discussed ideas.
Rescheduling: Arranging for another session if needed.	Provides additional counseling opportunities.
Termination of session: Offering appropriate generalizations from counseling to the client's outside world when goals have been achieved.	Brings counseling outcomes to the real world.
Evaluation of session: Asking the client to reflect on the essentials of each interview: "What will you take from today's session that will assist you between now and our next meeting?"	Provides tangible counseling outcomes for the client and counselor.
Follow-up: Connecting with the client about previous sessions, topics, and homework assignments.	Allows for continuity between counseling sessions.

Professionalism

SKILL AND DEFINITION	INTENTION
Developmental level match: Assessing the client's developmental level and selecting counseling interventions accordingly.	Creates intentional responses corresponding to client needs.
Ethics: Following a set of ethical guidelines provided by a professional organization; making appropriate ethical decisions.	Assists in remaining prudent in the decision-making process.
Professionalism: Making appropriate professional decisions following unwritten and written organizational mores and guidelines.	Adds respect to counselor and client.

RESOURCE B

Microskill Classification	Transcript of Rachel and Lori
	1. RACHEL: Honey, what could you possibly have to offer? You are a child with very little life experience, and you will never be able to help or understand my problems.
Minimal encourager	2. LORI: (nods and listens)
Pacing	3. RACHEL: How could you ever help me?
Paraphrase Open-ended question	4. LORI: Rachel, you are probably correct. I have not lived as long as you, and I don't have as much life experience as you. All I can do is listen to you and see if a counseling relationship develops. How does that sound to you?
	5. RACHEL: (finally sits down) It sounds fine, but it won't do any good. You see John and I were happily married for 50 years! He died quite suddenly six months ago, and I just don't know what to do.
Reflection of meaning and empathy/rapport	6. LORI: Having your husband be an important part of your life for so long and die unexpectedly must be devastating. I am very sorry.
	7. RACHEL: (pausing and looking at me) Do you have any idea what this is like?
Self-disclosure	8. LORI: I truly don't know what it is like to lose a husband, but I do know what it is like to lose a loved one; my father died when I was 25. I was scared and very sad.
	9. RACHEL: You are right, it is not the same, but at least you know some of what it feels like.
Reflection of meaning/ goal setting	10. LORI: So we have a few things in common, and one of your concerns we could work on in counseling is about the loss of your husband. Is that right?
	11. RACHEL: Yes, I would like to work on that, and I guess I'd like to talk about what to do with myself now that John is gone. We did so much together; it is like my left arm has been cut off.
Paraphrasing/reflection of meaning/pacing	12. LORI: Having John gone hits you at many different levels. Not only was he your companion with whom you did everything, it is also like a piece of you is missing as well.
	13. RACHEL: Yes, yes. There are many different levels. All three of our children are grown, but they so miss their dad *and* now they are calling me constantly to see if I am all right. Honestly, they are driving me crazy with their questions and concern! My youngest wants me to leave our home and move away with him.
Behavioral description/ leading	14. LORI: Rachel, I noticed that when you began talking of your children, your voice became higher and louder; you almost seemed agitated. Tell me more about your children and your relationship.
	15. RACHEL: I love my children, but we all have our own lives. It feels like now they suddenly think I am incapable of living by myself. I am only 71 years old! I still drive my car; I play duplicate bridge; I tutor first graders in reading . . . well, I mean I used to do those things.
Summarization	16. LORI: Let me see if I am truly understanding the situation. You miss your husband very much and are lonely, but recently your three children are trying to coddle you and even persuade you to possibly move away and live with them. You believe you are quite capable of living on your

Microskill Classification	Transcript of Rachel and Lori
	own without John, as you *used* to do many independent things. Many activities you and John did together, but some of these things sound as if you even did them without John. Am I correctly understanding the gist of it all?
	17. RACHEL: Yes, yes. (Rachel became silent again; I sat quietly with her for several very long minutes.) I miss the things John and I used to do! I miss my old life.
Verbal tracking/open-ended question/exploration/ understanding of concerns	18. LORI: Rachel, what do you miss about your old life?
	19. RACHEL: We were both retired, so we had the freedom to travel. We went everywhere. I have so many memories of our travels and years together. We have many friends in this town and throughout the country.
Reflection of meaning/ exploration/understanding of concerns	20. LORI: Those memories serve as a reminder of the great times together but they also remind you of your losses. Rachel, how many of those friends have you contacted recently?
	21. RACHEL: I received hundreds of cards and memorials. I answered each one with a hand-written thank-you note. But, I have not contacted anyone for a get-together since John's death.
Interpretation/paraphrase/ appropriate closed question perception check	22. LORI: Your loneliness goes deeper than John. Am I close?
	23. RACHEL: (crying) I miss my entire old life.
Reflection of feeling	24. LORI: The sadness and loss seems overwhelming.
	25. RACHEL: I don't know what to do.
Leading/teaching/special technique	26. LORI: Rachel, you have gone through six very difficult months. Even in this office you have exhibited many varying emotions, from shock to sadness to anger. These are very similar to the stages of grief. Your feelings are very normal and valid. The consequences of John's death seem to have shattered your old life. Let's set up several counseling goals to help you restructure your life and feelings.
	27. RACHEL: I wouldn't even know what goals to set.
Goal setting	28. LORI: You have already offered me several ideas, and there are many alternative ways to start. The first goal is to openly share your grief with others. You have done a wonderful job in here just by telling me your varying feelings and thoughts. I would like you to be this specific with your three children as well. Between now and our next session, you need to contact each of your children, telling them how you miss John and their dad and also how you feel about their coddling.
	29. RACHEL: Yes, I will call each child.
Goal setting/appropriate closed question	30. LORI: The only other goal I would like us to set today is that you will contact one of your duplicate bridge friends to find out the next arranged game time. Are you willing to do that?
	31. RACHEL: (smiles slowly) I am not sure about that one, but I will try.
Summarization of content and feeling	32. LORI: We have about 15 minutes left in our session. We have covered a lot of territory in our short time. I think I understand the depth of your loss. John must have been a great

(continued)

RESOURCE B CONTINUED

Microskill Classification	Transcript of Rachel and Lori
	partner. You miss him so much, and you are lonely. You would like to have your old life back. Topping it all off are your children who love you very much and are very concerned about you living alone. I have also learned you have given up much of what you used to enjoy such as bridge, tutoring, and traveling.
	33. RACHEL: We did cover a lot of territory. Until we started talking, I didn't realize how much I have lost.
Open-ended question/ evaluation of session	34. LORI: What part of the counseling session helps you understand why you have been so sad?
	35. RACHEL: Lots of things help me understand, but I am still somewhat confused.
Clarification/evaluation of session	36. LORI: Rachel, let's clarify even more then. What did we work on today that makes sense to you?
	37. RACHEL: Well, what I said earlier about not just John's dying, but I am sad about losing so much of my previous life.
Review of plan	38. LORI: You are sad about many of your losses, and today you stated that you are willing to regain control of at least two areas in your life. You will let your children know you love them but are very capable of living alone *and* you said you would call a duplicate bridge friend.
	39. RACHEL: I did say that, didn't I?!
Immediacy/ open-ended question	40. LORI: Yes, you did! I took from today's session that your feelings and grief are, indeed, valid and very normal. Rachel, you came here today very hesitant, and when you saw me, you knew I couldn't be of help.
Feedback/ evaluation of session	How are you feeling about us now?
	41. RACHEL: I still think you are very young. But you said you would listen and you did. Thank you, my dear child.
Open-ended question/ rescheduling	42. LORI: Rachel, it was a pleasure to work with you. What would you like to do about setting up another appointment?
	43. RACHEL: Could we meet the same time next week?
Pacing/termination of session	44. LORI: Let's check. That looks like an open time. Thanks, Rachel.

RESOURCE C

Counseling Interview Rating Form

Counselor: _____ Date: _____

Observer: _____ Tape Number: _____

Observer: _____ Audio or video (please circle)

Supervisor: _____ Session Number: _____

For each of the following specific criteria demonstrated, make a frequency marking every time the skill is demonstrated. Then assign points for consistent skill mastery using the ratings scales below. Active mastery of each skill receives a score of 2. Skills marked with an X should be seen consistently on every tape. List any observations, comments, strengths and weaknesses in the space provided. Providing actual counselor phrases is helpful when offering feedback.

Ivey Mastery Ratings

3 Teach the skill to clients (teaching mastery only)
2 Use the skill with specific impact on client (active mastery)
1 Use and/or identify the counseling skill (basic mastery)
   To receive an A on a tape, at least 52–58 points must be earned.
   To receive a B on a tape, at least 46–51 points must be earned.
   To receive a C on a tape, at least 41–45 points must be earned.

Specific Criteria		Frequency	Comments	Skill Mastery Rating
A. Opening/Developing Rapport				
1. Greeting	X			
2. Role definition/expectation				
3. Administrative tasks				
4. Beginning	X			
B. Exploration Phase/ Defining the Problem Microskills				
1. Empathy/rapport				
2. Respect				
3. Nonverbal matching	X			
4. Minimal encourager	X			
5. Paraphrasing	X			
6. Pacing/leading	X			
7. Verbal tracking	X			
8. Reflect feeling	X			
9. Reflect meaning	X			
10. Clarifications				
11. Open-ended questions				
12. Summarization	X			

(continued)

RESOURCE C CONTINUED

Specific Criteria		Frequency	Comments	Skill Mastery Rating
13. Behavioral description	X			
14. Appropriate closed question	X			
15. Perception check	X			
16. Silence	X			
17. Focusing	X			
18. Feedback	X			
C. Problem-Solving Skills/ Defining Skills				
1. Definition of goals	X			
2. Exploration/understanding of concerns	X			
3. Development/evaluation of alternatives	X			
4. Implement alternative				
5. Special techniques				
6. Process counseling				
D. Action Phase/Confronting Incongruities				
1. Immediacy				
2. Self-disclosure				
3. Confrontation				
4. Directives				
5. Logical consequences				
6. Interpretation				
E. Closing/Generalization				
1. Summarization of content/ feeling	X			
2. Review of plan	X			
3. Rescheduling				
4. Termination of session				
5. Evaluation of session	X			
6. Follow-up	X			
F. Professionalism				
1. Developmental level match				
2. Ethics				
3. Professional (punctual, attire, etc.)				
G. Strengths				
Area(s) for improvement				

Total _____

RESOURCE D

Counseling Interview Rating Form

Counselor: <u>Lori Russell-Chapin</u> Date: <u>6/28/04</u>

Observer: _____ Tape number: <u>1</u>

Observer: _____ Audio or video (please circle)

Supervisor: <u>Allen Ivey</u> Session Number: <u>Initial</u>

For each of the following specific criteria demonstrated, make a frequency marking every time the skill is demonstrated. Then assign points for consistent skill mastery using the ratings scales below. Active mastery of each skill receives a score of 2. Skills marked with an X should be seen consistently on every tape. List any observations, comments, strengths and weaknesses in the space provided. Providing actual counselor phrases is helpful when offering feedback.

Ivey Mastery Ratings

3   Teach the skill to clients (teaching mastery only)
2   Use the skill with specific impact on client (active mastery)
1   Use and/or identify the counseling skill (basic mastery)
    To receive an A on a tape, at least 52–58 points must be earned.
    To receive a B on a tape, at least 46–51 points must be earned.
    To receive a C on a tape, at least 41–45 points must be earned.

Specific Criteria		Frequency	Comments	Skill Mastery Rating
A. Opening/Developing Rapport				
1. Greeting	X			
2. Role definition/ expectation				
3. Administrative tasks				
4. Beginning	X			
B. Exploration phase/ defining the problem Microskills				
1. Empathy/rapport		I	"I am very sorry."	2
2. Respect				
3. Nonverbal matching	X			
4. Minimal encourager	X	I	(Nods.)	2
5. Paraphrasing	X	I	"Having John gone hits you at many different levels."	2

(continued)

RESOURCE D CONTINUED

Specific Criteria		Frequency	Comments	Skill Mastery Rating
6. Pacing/leading	X	II	"Rachel, you are probably correct."	2
7. Verbal tracking	X	III	"What do you miss about your old life?"	2
8. Reflect feeling	X	III	"You are lonely."	2
9. Reflect meaning	X	III	"Having your husband be an important part of your life for so long and die unexpectedly must be devastating."	2
10. Clarifications				
11. Open-ended questions		IIII	"How does that sound to you?"	2
12. Summarization	X	II	"Let me see if I truly understand the situation."	2
13. Behavioral description	X	I	"I noticed that when you began talking about your children, your voice became higher and louder . . . "	2
14. Appropriate closed question	X	III	"Am I close?" 2	
15. Perception check	X	III	"Is that right?"	2
16. Silence	X	I	(Listening.)	2
17. Focusing	X	I	"Between now and our next session, you need to contact each of your children telling them how . . . you feel about their codding."	2
18. Feedback	X	I	"Rachel, you came here today very hesitant . . ."	2
C. Problem-Solving Skills/Defining Skills				
1. Definition of goals	X	II	"The first goal is to openly share your grief with others."	2
2. Exploration/ understanding of concerns	X	II	"How many of those friends have you contacted lately?"	2
3. Development/ evaluation of alternatives	X	I	"There are many alternative ways to start."	2
4. Implement alternative				
5. Special techniques				
6. Process counseling		II	"Today you stated that you are willing to regain control of at least. . . ."	2
D. Action Phase/ Confronting Incongruities				
1. Immediacy		II	"How are you feeling about us now?"	2
2. Self-disclosure		I	"My father died when I was 25."	2
3. Confrontation				
4. Directives		I	" . . . you will contact one of your duplicate bridge friends . . . "	2

Specific Criteria		Frequency	Comments	Skill Mastery Rating
5. Logical consequences		I	"The consequences of John's death seem to have shattered your old life."	2
6. Interpretation		I	"Your loneliness goes deeper than John."	2
E. Closing/Generalization				
1. Summarization of content/feeling	X	I	"We did cover a lot of territory."	2
2. Review of plan	X	I	" . . . today you stated that you are willing . . . "	2
3. Rescheduling		I	"What would you like to do about setting up another appointment?"	2
4. Termination of session				
5. Evaluation of session	X	II	"What did we work on today that makes sense to you?"	2
6. Follow-up	X			
F. Professionalism				
1. Developmental level match		I	Assessing Rachel's developmental level as a 1 or 2.	2
2. Ethics				
3. Professional (punctual, attire, etc.)				

G. Strengths
  1. I liked the way you were able to build rapport with Rachel using the microcounseling skills and going with her resistance.
  2. The intentional use of reflections of feeling and meaning seemed to assist Rachel in better understanding her sadness.

H. Areas for Improvement
  1. Be cautious about asking too many opened and closed questions.
  2. Let Rachel brainstorm more ideas for grieving such as creating a memorial for John, etc.
  3. Even though Rachel read the Service Agreement describing confidentiality, be sure to discuss it next time.

Total: 58

RESOURCE E

Counseling Interview Rating Form	
Counselor: _____	Date: _____
Observer: _____	Tape Number: _____
Observer: _____	Audio or video (please circle)
Supervisor: _____	Session Number: _____

For each of the following specific criteria demonstrated, make a frequency marking every time the skill is demonstrated. Then assign points for consistent skill mastery using the ratings scales below. Active mastery of each skill receives a score of 2. Skills marked with an X should be seen consistently on every tape. List any observations, comments, strengths and weaknesses in the space provided. Providing actual counselor phrases is helpful when offering feedback.

Ivey Mastery Ratings

3   Teach the skill to clients (teaching mastery only).
2   Use the skill with specific impact on client (active mastery).
1   Use and/or identify the counseling skill (basic mastery).
     To receive an A on a tape, at least 52–58 points must be earned.
     To receive a B on a tape, at least 46–51 points must be earned.
     To receive a C on a tape, at least 41–45 points must be earned.

Specific Criteria		Frequency	Comments	Skill Mastery Rating
A. Opening/Developing Rapport				
1. Greeting	X			
2. Role definition/ expectation				
3. Administrative tasks				
4. Beginning	X			
B. Exploration Phase/ Defining the Problem Microskills				
1. Empathy/rapport				
2. Respect				
3. Nonverbal matching	X			
4. Minimal encourager	X			
5. Paraphrasing	X			
6. Pacing/leading	X			
7. Verbal tracking	X			
8. Reflect feeling	X			
9. Reflect meaning	X			
10. Clarifications				

Specific Criteria		Frequency	Comments	Skill Mastery Rating
11. Open-ended questions				
12. Summarization	X			
13. Behavioral description	X			
14. Appropriate closed question	X			
15. Perception check	X			
16. Silence	X			
17. Focusing	X			
18. Feedback	X			
C. Problem-Solving Skills/ Defining Skills				
1. Definition of goals	X			
2. Exploration/understanding of concerns	X			
3. Development/evaluation of alternatives	X			
4. Implement alternative				
5. Special techniques				
6. Process counseling				
D. Action Phase/Confronting Incongruities				
1. Immediacy				
2. Self-disclosure				
3. Confrontation				
4. Directives				
5. Logical consequences				
6. Interpretation				
E. Closing/Generalization				
1. Summarization of content/feeling	X			
2. Review of plan	X			
3. Rescheduling				
4. Termination of session				
5. Evaluation of session				
6. Follow-up	X			
F. Professionalism				
1. Developmental level match				
2. Ethics				
3. Professional (punctual, attire, etc.)				

G. Strengths

H. Areas for Improvement

Total _____

BECOMING EFFECTIVE AS A SUPERVISEE: THE INFLUENCE OF PLACEMENT SETTING

⇨ *You can only take your clients as far as you have gone yourself.*

OVERVIEW

GOALS

KEY CONCEPTS: YOU AND SUPERVISION

DETERMINING WHICH SUPERVISION STYLE WORKS BEST FOR YOU
DEVELOPMENTAL STYLES OF SUPERVISION
PRACTICAL REFLECTIONS 1: THE BEST FIT SUPERVISORY STYLES
PRACTICAL REFLECTIONS 2: PREFERRED MATURITY DIMENSIONS
PRACTICAL REFLECTIONS 3: CURRENT SUPERVISORY EXPECTATIONS

YOU AND YOUR SUPERVISION SETTING
SCHOOL SETTINGS
PRIMARY, MIDDLE, AND HIGH SCHOOLS
THE CASE OF STEPHEN
PRACTICAL REFLECTION 4: SCHOOL COUNSELING SUPERVISORY NEEDS

COLLEGES AND UNIVERSITIES
COMMUNITY AGENCIES
PRIVATE PRACTICE
HOSPITAL-BASED TREATMENT PROGRAMS
PRACTICAL REFLECTION 5: INFLUENCES OF FIELD EXPERIENCE SETTINGS

COLLECTING AND SHARING NEEDED INFORMATION
PRACTICAL REFLECTION 6: STUDENT PRACTICUM/INTERNSHIP AGREEMENT

EVALUATION OF YOUR WORK IN THE PLACEMENT SETTING
PRACTICAL REFLECTION 7: EVALUATION CONCERNS

SUMMARY AND PERSONAL INTEGRATION
PRACTICAL REFLECTION 8: INTEGRATION

REFERENCES
RESOURCES F THROUGH M

OVERVIEW

This chapter introduces you to effective supervision and the influences your placement settings may have on the structure, amount, and type of supervision available. You need to be knowledgeable enough about the supervisory process to assist the supervisor in the efficacy of the supervision process. You will learn about which supervision style matches your personal preferences and the special counseling considerations and implications that certain placement settings bring. The Case of Stephen is introduced, illustrating the unique needs a school setting may bring. The importance of supervision evaluation and its impact on you is stressed.

GOALS

1. Assess personal preferences for the differing dimensions of supervision.
2. Take responsibility for individual supervision needs.
3. Understand the unique supervision needs and skills of the settings of community agencies, schools, private practice, and hospital-based treatment programs.
4. Share forms and contracts establishing clear expectations for you, the agency, and the client.
5. Understand the need for evaluation and its benefits.

KEY CONCEPTS: YOU AND SUPERVISION

Supervision: A distinctive manner of approach and response to a supervisee's needs.

There are many differing dimensions of effective supervision. It is an area that has been the focus of much research from theoretical perspectives to outcome results. More about the theoretical models of supervision and further information on counseling outcome research will be discussed later in the text, but for the purposes of getting you started in supervision, five different aspects for becoming an effective supervisee will be addressed.

As you read this chapter, work hard at assessing honestly what you desire out of supervision and what your needs and expectations are from your supervisor. These ideas should be correlated with the goals, expectations, and counseling baseline from Chapters 1 and 2. Read each section and write down your preferences and self-acknowledgements. If you are willing to address these issues, you will have a very successful and power-ful supervision experience. The five areas for this chapter are determining which supervisory style works for you, discerning the unique influences of your placement setting, collecting and sharing needed information from your placement setting, understanding the supervision evaluation, and adjusting attitudinal perspectives.

DETERMINING WHICH SUPERVISION STYLE WORKS BEST FOR YOU

Supervision style is often very individual and very different. A basic defini-tion of supervision style suggests that it is a distinctive manner of approach and response to supervisees' needs (Friedlander & Ward, 1984). There is some outcome research on what makes effective supervision, and yet it is an area of much uncharted territory. It appears that there is not one clear-cut style of supervision that is best for everyone. It may be up to you, the student supervisee, to understand the varied dimensions of the supervi-sory process to assist in building the best situation for your supervisory experience. As each aspect of supervision is presented, you need to be looking for the best match of supervision dimensions for you.

At the end of this chapter in Resource F is a Supervisory Style Inven-tory (SSI) (Friedlander & Ward, 1984). You may want to take the inven-tory now, or read through this chapter and then take the SSI. Regardless of when you take the SSI, your results will help you to better under-stand what will make supervision more effective for you based on your preferences.

Developmental Styles of Supervision

Developmental supervision stages: supervisees progress through a series of pre-dictable levels or stages as they learn the skills of the counseling process.

There is much in the literature about the developmental nature of super-vision. The two major assumptions in developmental supervision are that you, the counselor in training, go through different developmental stages depending on your supervision needs. Secondly, just as you would assess the developmental level of your client in individual counseling, your su-pervision developmental level would be assessed and would require differ-ing types of supervisory responses (Stoltenberg, McNeill, & Delworth, 1998). One way to think about your developmental level is to focus on your experience and knowledge.

Hersey, Blanchard, and Johnson (2000) expanded that concept by di-viding your developmental or maturity level into four differing styles: structured, encouraging, coaching, and mentoring. Again for each level of developmental maturity or each differing situation you present, your supervisor will respond accordingly. In the Maturity Stage 1(M1), you might tell your supervisor that you don't know exactly what to do with a particular client. A M1 structured supervisory response may be to explain in detail what to do, "Try utilizing those basic interviewing skills. During the next interview, please use at least three reflections of feeling and meaning."

In the M2 stage, you may tell your supervisor that you are working with a client and you were able to conceptualize the case and necessary treatment interventions. A M2 encouraging supervisory response is, "You have worked hard on this case and thought it out thoroughly; I like how you stated your treatment goals."

In the M3 stage, you are excited to share the details on the case and request additional ideas. A M3 coaching supervisory response may sound like, "Using the intentional skill of self-disclosure seemed to work, but have you thought about how it changed the focus of the session?" In the final stage, M4, you tell your supervisor in a confident manner how the case is developing. You have very few questions. A M4 mentoring supervisory response is, "It is fun to share cases and hear how others intervene."

Other supervision theorists believe there are varying approaches to supervision such as either expressive or instrumental (Russo, 1993). Supervisors who use expressive approaches tend to be extraverts, enjoy people and relationships, and easily build rapport. Expressive supervisors tend to focus on how you are interacting with your clients and supervisors. An expressive response may sound like, "You seem very comfortable with your clients, and your warm and friendly demeanor puts people at ease." Those supervisors who prefer instrumental approaches tend to be introverts, encourage outcomes and goal setting, and be comfortable handling conflict in general. An instrumental supervisory response may be, "I noticed that you used open-ended questions when exploring your client's concerns, but when your client began to openly cry, you quickly asked a closed question and did not focus on the emotions. Next time you need to be willing to let your client sob."

Another supervision variable, according to Ladany, Marotta, and Muse-Burke (2001) is as trainees gain general experience, they become more adept at conceptualizing clients. In their research, the Supervisory Style Inventory (SSI) was administered to supervisees measuring students' perceptions of their supervisors. One of the outcomes of the research was that trainees preferred supervisors who were moderately high on all three styles: attractive, interpersonally sensitive, and task oriented.

Attractive supervisors are seen as warm, supportive, and often friendly. *Interpersonally sensitive supervisors* are seen as invested in the therapeutic process and what was happening to you the student, and the *task-oriented supervisor* is seen as providing structure to the supervision session and focusing on goals and task (Friedlander & Ward, 1984).

Practical Reflection 1: The Best Fit Supervisory Styles

Based on what you know about yourself, what style of supervision best fits your current supervision needs in the areas of attractiveness, interpersonal sensitivity, and task orientation? What were the results of your SSI?

_____

_____

_____

_____

Practical Reflection 2: Preferred Maturity Dimensions

Of the situational/maturity dimensions mentioned, list any supervision aspects that you prefer now such as structure, encouragement, coaching, or mentoring.

_____

_____

_____

_____

Practical Reflection 3: Current Supervisory Expectations

What are your expectations currently about supervisions? List them here and be sure to share with your supervisors.

_____

_____

_____

_____

YOU AND YOUR SUPERVISION SETTING

Now that you have a better understanding of some of the styles involved in supervision, you must be able to comprehend how your placement site may influence the type of supervision you receive. As each supervisor is different and unique, so is the actual placement site. Notice these differences, but look for some similar features that will illustrate consistency across professions. You and your fellow students will have practicum and internship experiences in a variety of settings, including schools, community agencies, hospitals, and private practice. Each setting, as well as the individuals and groups served, has unique needs and special opportunities for your counseling growth.

School Settings

Primary, Middle, and High Schools. In both public and private schools, as a school intern you will provide a variety of typically short-term, developmental academic, career, and social/personal counseling to students. Group counseling, parent and teacher consultation, and crisis intervention are among the more common services performed.

University and Community College. In college and university settings, you will gain experience in individual and group counseling, as well as outreach programming, crisis intervention, and academic counseling and development. Many counseling centers have several helping professionals on staff and work closely with student services, such as residence life and health services, to provide for the mental health needs of both traditional- and nontraditional-age students.

Primary, Middle, and High Schools

The school counselors' roles continue to change. You may become more focused on developmental education and the mental health needs of the school community as well as administrative opportunities. At some schools, the counselor intern may be the only mental health professional on site, while at others, the intern is part of a system that may include school counselors, school social workers, school psychologists, and student assistance program (SAP) professionals. These SAP professionals are often outside, contracted providers. Private schools may provide an even broader opportunity for developing a school counseling program. At each school level, the intern must become familiar with the developmental needs of the age group concerned and appropriate programs and interventions.

Supervision.   For school counselor interns, a credentialed school counselor must conduct the supervision. Be sure to check with your state board of education to understand the credentialing procedures in your state. Sometimes when there may be only one school counselor per school district who works with a number of different schools, locating a supervisor is a challenge. Many school counseling interns do not have a site supervisor located in the same building and is therefore not as readily accessible as at other sites. Although the intern may have an administrative supervisor on site such as the school principal, it is vital to be assertive about asking for and getting the support necessary on site. In cases where site supervision may not be as effective as desired, the university supervisor and group supervision with fellow students becomes more important. Interns should attempt to improve the on-site situation with their on-site supervisor and involve the university supervisor as necessary. Some schools will not have an office readily available for the counselor intern's use. Basic needs for the counselor intern are a space that provides for privacy and the ability to keep the client's visit confidential. Without this, school-age clients will not feel comfortable voluntarily seeking out the school counselor.

For all settings where the site supervisor is not directly on site, and in all school settings, interns should make themselves aware of emergency procedures. Schools should have crisis plans and perhaps even crisis teams to put into action when necessary. Many schools team with community agencies that can provide additional support to the school when necessary. Emergency procedures for reporting child abuse are also needed. Understand your state's laws and regulations for mandated reporting of sexual and child abuse.

Colleagues.   Many school counselors find themselves as "one of a kind" in their work setting, making networking through school counselors in the district and beyond, as well as through professional organizations a necessity to avoid isolation. Although colleagues are many, both the lack of understanding of what school counselors do and issues of confidentiality can lead to feelings of isolation as well. One of our group of three school counseling interns maintain monthly meetings five years after graduation, finding the resulting support and peer supervision invaluable in their roles as school counselors. Another networking system may be the use of the Internet and e-mail. You can use the International Counselor Network at <u>LISTSERVE@UTKVM1.UTK.EDU</u> to find colleagues online who can support your efforts and discuss related concerns. Obviously you would need to be discrete when discussing problems by avoiding names and other identifying references due to the nonconfidential nature of the Internet.

Clients.   In school settings, the clients might be students, parents, teachers, or groups of students. Counselor interns will get referrals from teachers who become aware of student concerns or behavior, from parents or guardians, the administration (particularly involving students with disciplinary problems), and from self-referrals. An intern in a school that did not previously have a school counselor will have to develop referral relationships and educate school members about all that school counselors can do, and in some cases, what they can't do! Basic forms and permissions will need to be devised, as well as policies and procedures for handling confidential material such as progress notes and intake information. The counseling emphasis will be short-term counseling aimed at assisting the student in learning ways to apply problem-solving skills to issues of concern. Opportunities for group counseling are many. School counselor interns have successfully run grief groups, social skills groups, academic improvement groups, play therapy groups, and even groups for parents. Consultation with teachers and parents is another major focus for the school counseling intern.

Confidentiality.   When working as a counselor with school-age children and in school settings, special legal and ethical considerations arise concerning confidentiality. School counselor interns should understand and implement the types of permission required by the school in which they work for students to be involved in individual and/or group counseling. Questions such as under what circumstances a child can see the school counselor without parent or guardian prior permission and what counseling records the parent or guardian has legal access to should be answered. Additionally, the intern and his or her site supervisor should address questions regarding what information can be released to referral sources such as teachers and administrators. Lawsuits have raised issues about counselor liability in circumstances such as suicide, drug abuse, abortion, and even success in college. School counselor interns need to be familiar with reporting procedures, duty to warn, and when to refer a student to community resources, among other responsibilities. It is essential that you obtain your own personal liability insurance. Many organizations offer student malpractice/liability insurance, including the American Counseling Association (ACA), American Mental Health Counseling Association (AMHCA), and National Association of Social Workers (NASW). Check to see if you are covered through your educational institution as well.

The Case of Stephen

As you read the Case of Stephen, begin to focus on the special needs that a school placement site may bring. Think about the supervision needs of Lori as she begins to understand the complexities of Stephen's counseling needs.

Stephen was referred to me during my days as a school counselor/school psychologist. I spent twenty hours a week as a school counselor in a rural Western town and the remaining twenty hours a week as a school psychologist for the same district administering tests and facilitating multi-disciplinary case study teams.

Stephen's mother was very upset as Stephen was falling behind in his studies and continuing to lose interest in his friends and his love for soccer.

Stephen's father committed suicide six months prior to my interviewing this eleven-year-old boy. His dad had been in a high-pressured administrative position, and the company had filed for bankruptcy. Stephen was the person to find his dad's body hanging in the family basement. This rural community had few mental health resources, but the family was seen by their church pastor immediately following the funeral.

You may want to follow along using a blank Counseling Interview Rating Form (CIRF), which was introduced in Chapter 2. Below is the second counseling interview between Stephen and me. To compare your scores with ours, see the completed CIRF in Resource G.

> LORI: *Stephen, it is good to see you again. What do you want to work on today?*
> STEPHEN: *(Silence.)*
> LORI: *(Silence.)*
> STEPHEN: *I don't want to work on anything. It is so boring in here.*
> LORI: *It is kind of boring in here. Let's go to the play therapy room.*
> STEPHEN: *That must be for babies, but it has to be better than here!*
> LORI: *(The play therapy room was two doors down.) Play with anything you want.*
> STEPHEN: *(He wandered around for several minutes and became intrigued with the small sand play area. Stephen picked up a large plastic dinosaur and began chasing the smaller dinosaurs.)*
> LORI: *Those smaller dinosaurs must be scared. The big one may feel pretty powerful and in control.*
> STEPHEN: *Yah.*
> LORI: *Stephen, when was the last time you felt powerful and in control?*
> STEPHEN: *I guess it was before my dad died. (A tear trickled slowly down his cheek.)*
> LORI: *Stephen, that must have been so scary and sad when your dad died. I am so sorry that your dad killed himself and felt he had no other options. I am sorry that you found you dad dead in the basement.*
> STEPHEN: *(Our eyes meet for the first time and both of us are crying.) It was awful! Why did he have to leave us?*

LORI: *(Silence.) I don't know, Stephen. It is important, though, that you begin talking about your thoughts and feelings surrounding your dad's suicide.*

STEPHEN: *I don't want to talk about it. It hurts too much.*

LORI: *(Silence.) Do you like to read?*

STEPHEN: *Sometimes.*

LORI: *Let's not talk then but read instead. I have a wonderful book called* The Hurt. *It is quite easy to read and probably too simple for you. Perhaps we could read it together and then you may want to tell the story to your younger brother, Abe.*

STEPHEN: *Whatever.*

LORI: *(We read the book together, alternating pages read out loud.) This is one of my favorite stories. What does it mean to you?*

STEPHEN: *It is a pretty good book. Abe would like it. He doesn't talk much either. It is a story about a little boy who stops talking about his hurt feelings. The hurt moves into his room. The little boy becomes more sad and lonely, and the hurt gets as big as his room.*

LORI: *That must be how Abe feels. I am guessing that may be how you feel too, Stephen!*

STEPHEN: *I guess it is.*

LORI: *Tell me what things you have tried to make your hurt go away.*

STEPHEN: *I have worked hard around our house helping my mom.*

LORI: *That must be a huge responsibility for the oldest man in your house.*

STEPHEN: *It is, but mom needs my help. She doesn't have anyone else.*

LORI: *So in order to be the man and maybe even take the place of your dad, you can't focus on your studies and fun things like soccer because you have so much to do around the house.*

STEPHEN: *I have lots to do and besides soccer is for kids.*

LORI: *The man of the house can't have fun anymore?*

STEPHEN: *Sure, I guess.*

LORI: *(I picked up an inflatable beach ball and threw it at Stephen. He caught it with a surprised look on his face.) Let's play ball for a while. Look where you caught the ball using your left thumb. What word is written on that section of the ball?*

STEPHEN: Hopeless.

LORI: *Talk to me about your hopeless feelings.*

STEPHEN: *Everything is hopeless. Nothing seems to get better. Everyone says time will make it better, but it hasn't.*

LORI: *Time alone is not healing your hurt. In fact it gets bigger by doing nothing.*

STEPHEN: *Maybe.*

LORI: *Let's keep throwing the ball. (I dropped it this time, so I picked it up strategically. My thumb happened to land on the word* devastated.*) One of the last times I was devastated was when my dad died. I was 25 years old, so older than you. I do remember, though, thinking my world had crumbled and feeling abandoned.*

STEPHEN: *Well, I bet you didn't have to see your dad hanging from a rope!*

LORI: *No, Stephen, I did not. I can't imagine how difficult that must have been.*

STEPHEN: *I tried to save him, you know.*

LORI: *I didn't know that.*

STEPHEN: *I got on a chair and cut him down with a knife we had. He fell to the floor. I thought maybe I killed him by the fall. I then tried helping him breathe like I had seen on TV.*

LORI: *You were very brave, Stephen.*

STEPHEN: *It didn't do much good, did it?*

LORI: *You couldn't save his life, but maybe you helped him in his death. What do you think your dad wants for you in his death?*

STEPHEN: *(Long pause.) He wants me to be happy.*

LORI: *What do you need to do to be happy and alive?*

STEPHEN: *I don't know.*

LORI: *Guess with me then.*

STEPHEN: *Have some fun. Study hard. Take care of Mom and Abe. Stuff.*

LORI: *Let's have some more fun here. I have one more game to play and then we will close up. Do you know the game of Tic, Tac, Toe?*

STEPHEN: *Sure.*

LORI: *You can draw the needed squares on this paper. Our goal is to work on your having more fun and studying harder. So every time you place an X, you must come up with one idea how to have fun and study harder. When I place my O, I will offer some ideas too. Go. (We played the game until the "cat" won and all the squares had been filled.)*

LORI: *Stephen, you have played and worked a lot in our time together. What will you take with you from our session today that you can use in the week to come?*

STEPHEN: *Well, this hasn't been as boring as I thought! I guess I learned that my hurt has gotten really big! I have to remember to tell Abe the story.*

Practical Reflection 4: School Counseling Supervisory Needs

What unique supervisory needs are presented with the Case of Stephen? Think about Stephen's age, school life, homework, family, and so on.

_____

_____

_____

_____

LORI: *Your hurt was really big. You were able today to make it much smaller by talking about your thoughts and feelings. Would you like to borrow the book to read to Abe?*

STEPHEN: *Sure. I will bring it back next week.*

LORI: *Stephen, thanks for working and playing with me. During the next week I need you to work and play again. What is one thing that you will work on and one thing that you will play?*

STEPHEN: *(He smiled at me.) I will turn in my science homework, and I will play with Abe.*

LORI: *Those two tasks sound important and even fun. When shall we make the next appointment?*

STEPHEN: *I could make it after my soccer practice next Wednesday.*

LORI: *See you then, Stephen. I hope Abe will like the book too.*

Colleges and Universities

Practicum and internship experience in the counseling center at a community college, college, or university offers a variety of opportunities ranging from crisis intervention to career development and counseling. Professional counselors and other mental health professionals who deal with the range of presenting concerns of college students, faculty, and administration staff the college or university counseling center. As a part of student affairs and/or student services, counseling center staff typically works closely with administrators and even faculty in dealing with the mental health needs on campus.

Supervision.   The counseling center director or his or her designee serves as site supervisor. If there are specialists in the center, such as a substance abuse counselor or eating disorders expert, the intern may seek their supervision concerning certain clients. Weekly staff meetings are usually held to discuss cases, plan programming efforts, deal with administrative matters, and share information regarding the types of clients and presenting concerns being encountered. As a community within the larger community, it is necessary to learn and communicate trends and issues with which students deal. Learning the intake process, limits of treatment provided, and referral sources are matters dealt with early on in supervision. The *intake process* entails learning to conduct a complete assessment in order to recommend treatment options. For some counseling centers, the intake process is separate from treatment, with the intake counselor recommending the most appropriate treatment provider within or outside of the counseling center. Many centers offer in-service education programs, as well as the opportunity to sit in on counseling sessions for observation.

Colleagues.   Professionals working in college counseling centers come from a variety of backgrounds, including social work, psychology, and counseling. Counseling centers may also use paraprofessionals and interns from various academic departments to provide services. Paraprofessionals can be students who are trained as peer counselors, providing information and support to students on a variety of issues and concerns. Counseling interns may have opportunities to be involved in training of paraprofessionals in helping skills. Colleagues may have developed certain areas of expertise that will be useful for consultation as you work with clients with a variety of presenting concerns.

Clients.   Clients in college and university counseling centers may range from the traditional age college freshmen experiencing being away from home for the first time, to the older international student seeking a degree far from home. Many adjustment problems come to the attention of counseling centers. Students may have difficulty adjusting to college life, residence hall life, new relationships, old relationships, family relationships, choosing a major or program of study, and career direction, among other issues. Other concerns typically dealt with in counseling centers include depression, eating disorders, substance abuse, and anxiety disorders. Occasionally, a serious mental illness such as schizophrenia emerges in late adolescence. Older adults returning to college or starting later than the traditional age may also experience concerns needing attention through the counseling center.

An important part of working in a counseling center is outreach programming. Interns develop teaching and presentation skills by providing information to groups of students about topics of interest and concern such as substance abuse, eating disorders, sexually transmitted diseases, and stress management. Presentations on academically-oriented topics such as time management, test anxiety, and study skills present opportunities to develop skills while providing important preventive services. Additionally, many students benefit from participation in group counseling, where topics can range from body image to career exploration. Counseling interns have found success in establishing such groups even in centers where group participation has not previously been offered or established.

Confidentiality. Although the limits of confidentiality are the same in counseling centers as in other settings, it can be difficult for students to seek services, fearing that others will consider them "crazy" if it is discovered they have visited the counseling center. Normalizing the process of seeking mental health services is a challenge to all professional counselors, and college and university counseling centers have worked toward this end. Outreach programming is one way that counseling centers provide students with information about services offered. Informally learning about the intake process and meeting a person who works as a counselor can alleviate some of the fear of using counseling services.

Those who refer students to the counseling center include faculty, residence hall personnel, family members, and others. Interns need to learn what is appropriate to share with referral sources, depending on the releases of consent signed, as well as university policy and legal status of the client. Educating referral sources about the importance of confidentiality and its limits also assists in the process.

Community Agencies

Community agencies provide diverse opportunities for counseling with special clients, ranging from agencies providing services for the elderly, victims of sexual assault and domestic violence, foster care and child welfare, to those with persistent mental illnesses and substance abuse problems. In many agencies, counselor interns work as part of a treatment team, along with psychiatrists, social workers, case managers and workers, as well as professionals from other agencies involved with a client. Additionally, in many cases, counselor interns may be working with the judicial system when their clients have court-mandated treatment obligations or are involved in legal matters. Individual, family, and group counseling, including in-home treatment, as well as psychoeducational programming, assessment, and case management activities, may all be part of the counselor intern's work at an agency.

Supervision. In community agencies, counselor interns may have a variety of opportunities for supervision in addition to the designated site supervisor. Many agencies have teams of service providers, and at team meetings, specific cases are presented for consultation, supervision, and information sharing. Valuable input can be gained from others working directly on the client's case as well as other team members. The case presentation format is useful in sharing necessary information about a client for others to assist and respond. At many agencies, a variety of professionals and paraprofessionals provide services, expertise and experiences to share with a counselor intern. Informal supervision may occur often during the day as the counselor intern seeks input from available colleagues. One of the challenges of working at a community agency is the paperwork necessary for documentation of services. Supervision will include getting feedback on the appropriate documentation of services according to funding and accrediting sources. It is important to build in time during working hours to complete documentation, whether written or dictated.

As at any site, counselor interns should learn what emergency procedures are on site. Examples of emergencies include a suicidal client, a client threatening violence, and potential danger at a home visit. Interns should be trained in procedures and emergency agency contacts when the site supervisor is not available.

Colleagues. After training and a certain amount of time spent at the agency, interns find themselves feeling and being treated as a full staff member. Colleagues will be from a variety of professional training backgrounds including psychology, social work, and human services, as well as counseling. Learning from each can add greatly to the internship experience. At agencies with residential settings, a variety of service providers work with clients around the clock. Communication among shifts is vital for continuity in treatment. Opportunities for continuing and in-service education are provided by many agencies; it is important to find out what is available and participate. Many agencies use volunteers in different capacities as well. As an intern, recognizing the value of and participating in the training and education of volunteers is an additional opportunity for professional development. Although you may find yourself being treated as a full member of the staff and find many opportunities for learning, remember to set limits on what you take on as an intern.

Clients. At community agencies, counselor interns work with clients in outpatient, residential, home-based, and/or community-based settings. You might work with an agency that serves victims of violence, the elderly, children and families, substance abuse, involuntary clients, clients involved with protective services, and any number of presenting concerns. Many agencies serve a specified clientele based on funding sources. For example, an agency serving elderly clients might only provide services to those over 65, or a children's agency may only serve those 18 years or younger. Other agencies are affiliated with a religious organization and may have restrictions on the types of services provided.

Many agencies provide counseling and mental health services to clients who are mandated or directed to seek treatment. A parent attempting to regain custody of a child might be court ordered to complete substance abuse treatment and/or parenting classes. A child or adult adjudicated in the legal system may be mandated for counseling as part of successfully completing probation. In these cases and others, clients may have a variety of feelings and responses to the counselor assigned. In addition, most clients in this situation will have signed a release of information for the counselor to report progress to the referring agent. Establishing a therapeutic relationship can be difficult under these circumstances. In the initial session, it is important to ask the client their feelings about the referral and reflect and acknowledge those feelings as legitimate. The client's negative feelings are usually directed at the referring source and, once acknowledged and legitimized, the counselor can move toward establishing some beginning trust in the relationship. When working with mandated clients, it is also necessary to discuss the limits of confidentiality with the referring source as well as the consequences for choosing not to follow through with counselor recommendations. For example, when working with clients on parole who are mandated for outpatient substance abuse treatment, clients should be asked what the consequences would be for choosing not to comply with treatment. When treatment is presented as a choice, and even though to choose not to comply meant violating parole, clients may feel more empowered about their choice for treatment.

Confidentiality.   The ethical obligation of protecting your client's right to confidentiality has certain limits within the context of working in community agencies, particularly in circumstances where the counselor intern is a mandated reporter. As a mandated reporter, counselor interns must report incidences of suspected physical or sexual abuse or neglect of children and the elderly to appropriate authorities. Counselors can become aware of abuse or neglect from primary sources and/or secondary sources. The limits of confidentiality should be stated so that all clients and their guardians understand under what circumstances the counselor must break confidentiality without client consent. The agency should have a standard form of informed consent that includes information regarding confidentiality of client information. When working with children, interns must know who is the legal guardian of the child because this is the person with legal right to the child's information. Client information may be shared between counselor intern and supervisor, and/or with other members of a treatment team within the agency without violating confidentiality. Clients should, however, be made aware of who will have access to their information.

An example is gaining client permission to videotape sessions for supervision or class assignments. Clients should be given explicit information about who will be viewing the tape, under what circumstances and for what purpose, and how the tape will be erased.

Private Practice

In private practice, one or more licensed professionals organize their own company to provide counseling services. These services may include individual, family, and group counseling as well as organizational consulting and Employee Assistance Programs. Although many private practices have set fees and clients use insurance coverage to help pay for services, some use a sliding fee scale, particularly for services provided by a counselor intern. Private practice settings may specialize in certain areas such as Christian Counseling or Court Evaluations; however, most offer comprehensive, generalist practice. Counselor interns in private practice settings typically are exposed to a diverse clientele with a variety of presenting concerns.

Supervision. In a private practice setting, there are several opportunities for supervision. Your supervisor might be a licensed psychologist, a licensed clinical social worker, a licensed professional clinical counselor, or even a psychiatrist. In each case, it is vital to understand the training and approach to counseling and psychotherapy that your supervisor has had. In addition to the one-on-one supervision of your site supervisor, you will typically be involved in staff meetings and group supervision meetings as well. You may find that you bring a different, perhaps more developmental perspective to the understanding of client concerns. Staff meetings will also include marketing, client service, and other aspects of maintaining and growing the practice. Training by individuals within the practice and opportunities to attend other training sessions may be available. If your supervisor is also the owner of the practice, you may have opportunities to be involved in development of the organization and its client base. Due to the nature of most private practices, your supervisor will typically be heavily involved in client services and may be limited to the one hour of weekly scheduled supervision time. Interns can make the most of supervision by being prepared with questions, reviewed tapes, and administrative concerns.

Colleagues. Practitioners who work in private practice come from many fields in the helping professions, including counselors, social workers, and psychologists, as well as pastoral counselors and others with Master's degrees who have met licensing standards. In some cases, these practitioners work under another's license such as the licensed psychologist's. For those insurance or managed care companies allowing this practice, interns might also work under this arrangement. Your colleagues will typically be working for a percentage of the fees they bring to the practice; for example, the practitioner receives 50 percent of the fees generated and 50 percent go to the practice for overhead expenses such as secretarial support, office rent, and equipment. In other cases, practitioners might work for the practice for an hourly wage, and, as an employee, have withholding taxes, liability insurance, and other expenses taken care of by the employer. With the working structure of a private practice, staff meetings or supervision usually structures time with colleagues. Occasionally, when clients cancel or do not show for an appointment, there is the opportunity for collegial visits.

Clients. For most practitioners and clients in private practice, the greatest challenge for providing service can be managed care. Managed care began as an effort to control skyrocketing costs of medical and mental health care and to provide some standardization of medical and mental health treatment protocols. Although in some ways managed care has met these goals, in many cases client treatment has changed dramatically and not always for the good. In the past, insurance companies may have covered unlimited numbers of sessions for mental health treatment. Presently, most companies require approval of services and documentation of treatment goals, progress, and success for services to be covered. Private practitioners apply to managed care companies to become network service providers. This process can take months, and the practitioner generally accepts a lower fee than usually charged to become a participating provider. Additionally, some companies limit the type of mental health provider who can provide treatment. Clients make choices for treatment and providers based on what managed care companies will approve. Many times the managed care company allows an assessment to determine what treatment is indicated. The managed care company might conduct the assessment, or an employee assistance program or other company contracted by the managed care company might be utilized. Recommendations are then made for the client's treatment and a suitable network provider is sought. Depending on the requirements of the managed care company, interns might not be deemed suitable for providing treatment, even under the supervision of the established provider.

One of the challenges for interns in a private practice is getting enough direct client counseling hours. Although there may be ample opportunity for psychoeducational presentations, pro bono work, and other supportive work such as administering and scoring tests, interns rarely have established referral sources for clients. Developing a referral base is essential for success; churches, physicians, other interns, and schools might be places to contact. A sliding fee scale for intern's services can also assist in establishing a client base. When potential clients are referred to the practice and can not afford regular fees, intern services at reduced fees can be a viable option for many.

Confidentiality.   As in community agencies, clients need to be informed what the limits of confidentiality are in a private practice. Additionally, clients must be informed as to who will see videotapes or hear audiotapes of the intern's counseling sessions. Many interns have difficulty asking clients to agree to be videotaped or audiotaped for supervision and course expectations. Informing the client as to the purpose of the tape, who specifically will see the tape, and how it will be disposed of can assist the client in agreeing to the request. It may also help to remind the client that, as a counselor in training, your supervisors and classmates provide valuable feedback for learning. Many an intern who has difficulty with clients agreeing to be taped, when asked about their approach, will have put the process in a negative light, thereby making it easier for the client to reject the request. Some clients will give consent if their back is to the camera and only the counselor intern's face can be seen. Although not ideal, it assists in learning to be able to gauge client reactions and nonverbal communication. This setup can work for most supervisees and supervisors. Children usually readily agree to taping and as long as the parent and/or legal guardian approves; it is helpful to get permission from the child as well. Letting the child see into the camera, view a few minutes of tape, and generally become comfortable with the process can assist in lessening the impact of taping when the session starts. A general discussion of how students have successfully videotaped will facilitate the process for those who are more hesitant.

Hospital-Based Treatment Programs

Hospitals provide mental health treatment programs on an inpatient, partial hospitalization, and outpatient basis. Programs range from eating disorders to attention deficit hyperactivity disorder (ADHD) clinics, to substance abuse, and may serve all age groups. Most hospital-based programs utilize group therapy as a primary treatment, particularly at the inpatient and partial hospitalization levels of treatment. Counselor interns will work with a variety of treatment providers including nurses, psychiatrists, psychologists, and social workers.

Supervision.   Higher numbers of professional counselors are being hired to work in hospital-based settings more often and in different capacities than ever before. Depending on the program the intern selects, the supervisor's training can range from psychiatry, to social work, to mental health nursing. A professional counselor's identity and niche are important in mental health treatment in hospital-based settings as treatment focus moves away from a strict medical model to a more holistic, even developmental model. Supervision may entail learning the supervisor's theoretical approach and foundation and sharing of the intern's emergent theoretical beliefs. If the program is inpatient or a partial hospitalization, opportunities for supervision may occur at several times throughout the day or week. Frequently, a team approach is used in treatment. During team meetings, client cases are discussed with each member of the team contributing ideas, impressions, information, and recommendations.

Colleagues.   As stated previously, colleagues and treatment team members come from a variety of training backgrounds. Interns may find themselves coleading a treatment group or other therapeutic interventions and disagreeing with the approach used by their colleague. Counseling interns may find themselves at odds with the approaches used by other professionals who may not have counseling training, yet are providing counseling services. Learning from each other is vital in improving services offered to clients. Interns should be open to learning from the experiences of others and willing to share what they have learned as well.

Clients.   Clients in hospital-based settings, particularly those in inpatient and partial hospitalization, are generally suffering more acute phases of mental disorders. Inpatient programs generally attempt to stabilize the client through medication and treatment, and then release the client to follow-up services in an outpatient or partial hospitalization program. The client will receive a diagnosis of their condition, possibly be involved with psychological testing, and receive group, individual counseling, or both, as part of their treatment. Additional services may include medical treatment, occupational therapy, and discharge planning. For some hospital-based treatment programs, a specific diagnosis or cluster of diagnoses are treated in a specialized program. Examples include substance dependence, eating disorders, and gambling addiction. Inpatient mental health treatment programs exist for children, adolescents, and adults.

Confidentiality.   Confidentiality can be challenging in inpatient and partial hospitalization programs as clients and staff members interact. Clients and even staff members who are always on duty when on the unit can also challenge boundaries. Generally, all treatment professionals who interact with clients chart the interaction so there is a record of all treatment the client receives. In this way, those who work other shifts and other treatment team members have information about what happened with the client while they were not present. Many interns have found hospital charting of progress notes to be different than what is required in an agency. An important part of training is learning what belongs on a client's chart, because it is the master record of the client's treatment while hospitalized.

Practical Reflection 5: Influences of
Field Experience Settings

How is your practicum and internship setting influencing your field experience and your supervision? Analyze this from the standpoints of supervision opportunities and structure, colleagues, clients, and confidentiality.

_____

_____

_____

_____

COLLECTING AND SHARING NEEDED INFORMATION

As you can see, the type of placement site does influence your counseling and supervisory experience. Another essential component of your overall experience is sharing information about you, once you have selected a placement setting. As soon as you have taken the opportunity to let your supervisor get to know who you are, we also hope you will ask your supervisor to share his or her collective wisdom. Learning about theoretical orientations and other's training experiences can be fun and interesting. Reciprocity is a treasured relationship builder.

We all fear that which we don't understand and is unknown, so you can alleviate some of that anxiety by letting your supervisor know as much relevant information about you as possible. If you have an updated resume, please make copies for your supervisor and instructor. Your field experience instructor may have special forms to assist you with sharing this information and other course requirements. If not, Resources H through M are provided so that you may use or adapt them. Several of the forms were adapted from classic materials developed by Dimick and Krause, (1980).

These forms and needed information may also assist your counseling program in following the necessary accreditation guidelines for field experience and supervision. Remember to use the forms your educational institution and agencies have first. The forms presented here are only examples for you to use if needed.

Two forms that protect you, your institution, and your placement site are the Student Practicum/Internship Agreement and the Practicum/

Practical Reflection 6: Student Practicum/ Internship Agreement

After looking at the Student Practicum/Internship Agreement, what other valuable information would you want to include? What might your instructor want you to include?

_____

_____

_____

_____

Internship Contract. The Student Practicum/Internship Agreement and an extra copy will assure all that you have read your professional code of ethics, you understand the policies of the professional organization, you have proof of student liability and malpractice insurance, and you agree with and understand the course expectations laid out before you (see Resource H for a sample form). Resource I is an example of a contract between the university and the actual field placement site clarifying the expectations and roles of each party.

These next few sample forms may be presented to you in a field experience packet. Regardless of the manner of distribution, please fill out each form or needed piece of information in a timely and comprehensive manner and be sure to share all with your supervisors, whether they be on site or your university instructor. Keep an extra copy of everything just in case some information gets lost!

Your packet may include a log sheet to help you in accurately and consistently collecting your weekly field experience hours (see Resource J for an example log sheet). Your instructor will let you know when to turn in your hours, but you need to find a method of habitually writing down your hours of direct and indirect service hours. *Direct service hours* are any counseling activity where you are actively and directly working with clients, such as individual and group counseling, educational workshops, and consultations where you are presenting materials. *Indirect service hours* are those where you are not directly responsible for the activity, but it is an essential part of your counseling responsibilities, such as case notes, client files, pertinent reading, supervision sessions, staffings, and class time. For many of you in accredited counseling programs, you must acquire a minimum of 700 clock hours for the entire field experience with at least 240 indirect hours. The specific breakdown is 100 hours for practicum and 600 hours for internship.

Two other important forms for you to become familiar with are a Client Informed Consent Form and a Client Release Form. These forms are essential to you, the intern counselor, and to the client; they clarify the counseling relationship and expectations. These forms must be signed and placed in your student file at the university and your personal student file to serve as added protection to you and the consumer of counseling services. The Client Informed Consent Form ensures that the client understands who you are and the extent of your counseling training. In addition it offers approval for videotaping of the session. The Client Release Form offers approval for you to counsel a child or minor, and it could also provide a place for you to share needed information with others. It is important to have the effective dates the contract begins and ends. Official institutional letterhead is essential for identification. Resources K and L are offered as examples, but your individual universities and settings may have similar forms developed for their unique population and settings.

EVALUATION OF YOUR WORK IN THE PLACEMENT SETTING

Earlier in the chapters, you have learned that true supervision will always include an evaluation component. It seems you are in a constant state of evaluation when receiving feedback on your weekly counseling tapes. In a manner of speaking you are, but there will be a formal evaluation, usually at a midpoint in the semester and at the end of the semester. Be sure to ask these important questions about the evaluations. How much are they worth point wise in proportion to your entire grade? Who will get to see them? Where do they go? When do you get to review the evaluation (Sweitzer & King, 1999)?

There are different types of evaluations, such as narratives and open-ended questions or Likert-type scales numbering from 1 to 6. Resource M is a sample Site Supervisor's Evaluation of Student Counselor's Performance that uses a Likert-type scale (Hackney & Nye, 1973). Notice the different categories used to examine your counseling competencies: supervision comments, the counseling process, the conceptualization process, and additional suggestions. Be sure to set up a special supervision session for your midterm evaluation or use a regularly scheduled appointment to review your evaluation. There is also a place for your signature and that of your supervisor. Review your supervisor's evaluation carefully and work on

Practical Reflection 7: Evaluation Concerns

What are your biggest concerns about the evaluation process? Talk among your classmates about their concerns.

---

areas that need improvement in the next time period. In many programs, students have the opportunity to evaluate the supervisor as well. This mechanism provides the supervisor with important information to improve his or her skills. If any problems arise that cannot be resolved between the supervisor and supervisee, the university instructor can act as a third-party mediator.

SUMMARY AND PERSONAL INTEGRATION

This Chapter outlines unique variables influencing your supervisory experience.

- In the section on Determining Which Supervisory Style Works for You, information was shared so you could select the best supervision match for your cognitive and emotional style of interviewing and counseling.
- In You and the Supervision Setting, each placement setting was presented listing special considerations, learning opportunities, and skill development.
- Sample forms and evaluations procedures were offered to assist you and your school and agency in gathering and sharing needed counseling information.
- The final section comprised attitudinal perspectives that may be strengths, but if not addressed could cause potential supervisory problems.

Practical Reflection 8: Integration

Which of the above supervisory dimensions will assist you most in becoming a productive and effective interviewer, counselor, and supervisee?

_____

_____

_____

_____

REFERENCES

Friedlander, M. L., & Ward, L. G. (1984). Development and validation of the Supervisory Styles Inventory. *Journal of Counseling Psychology, 31*, 541–57.

Dimick, K.M. & Krause, F.H. (1980). (4th ed.). Practicum Manual for Counseling and Psychotherapy. Muncie, IN: Accelerated Development Inc.

Hackney, H. & Nye, S. (1973). Counseling Strategies and Objectives. Upper Saddle River, NJ: Prentice-Hall.

Hersey, P., Blanchard, K., & Johnson, D. (2000). *Management of Organizational Behavior: Leading Human Resources* (8th ed.). Upper Saddle River, NJ: Prentice Hall.

Ladany, N., Marotta, S., & Muse-Burke, J. (2001). Counselor experience related to complexity of case conceptualization and supervision preference. *Counselor Education and Supervision, 40*, 203–19.

Russo, J. R. (1993). *Serving and Surviving as a Human Service Worker* (2nd ed.). Prospect Heights, IL: Waveland Press.

Stoltenberg, C. D., McNeill, B., & Delworth, U. (1998). *IDM Supervision, An Integrated Developmental Model for Supervising Counselors and Therapists*. San Francisco: Jossey-Bass.

Sweitzer, H. F., & King, M. (1999). *The Successful Internship: Transformation and Empowerment*. Pacific Grove, CA: Brooks/Cole.

A special thank you to Dr. Nancy Sherman who wrote this chapter's section on supervision placement sites.

RESOURCE F

Supervisory Styles Inventory*

For trainees' form: Please indicate your perception of the style of your current or most recent supervisor of psychotherapy/counseling on each of the following descriptors. Circle the number on the scale, from 1 to 7, which best reflects your view of him or her.

For supervisors' form: Please indicate your perceptions of your style as a supervisor of psychotherapy/counseling on each of the following descriptors. Circle the number on the scale, from 1 to 7, which best reflects your view of yourself.

	NOT VERY						VERY
1. Goal oriented	1	2	3	4	5	6	7
2. Perceptive	1	2	3	4	5	6	7
3. Concrete	1	2	3	4	5	6	7
4. Explicit	1	2	3	4	5	6	7
5. Committed	1	2	3	4	5	6	7
6. Affirming	1	2	3	4	5	6	7
7. Practical	1	2	3	4	5	6	7
8. Sensitive	1	2	3	4	5	6	7
9. Collaborative	1	2	3	4	5	6	7
10. Intuitive	1	2	3	4	5	6	7
11. Reflective	1	2	3	4	5	6	7
12. Responsive	1	2	3	4	5	6	7
13. Structured	1	2	3	4	5	6	7
14. Evaluative	1	2	3	4	5	6	7
15. Friendly	1	2	3	4	5	6	7
16. Flexible	1	2	3	4	5	6	7
17. Prescriptive	1	2	3	4	5	6	7
18. Didactic	1	2	3	4	5	6	7
19. Thorough	1	2	3	4	5	6	7
20. Focused	1	2	3	4	5	6	7
21. Creative	1	2	3	4	5	6	7
22. Supportive	1	2	3	4	5	6	7
23. Open	1	2	3	4	5	6	7
24. Realistic	1	2	3	4	5	6	7
25. Resourceful	1	2	3	4	5	6	7
26. Invested	1	2	3	4	5	6	7

*Developed by M. L. Friedlander and L. G. Ward (1984).   *(continued)*

RESOURCE F CONTINUED

27. Facilitative	1	2	3	4	5	6	7
28. Therapeutic	1	2	3	4	5	6	7
29. Positive	1	2	3	4	5	6	7
30. Trusting	1	2	3	4	5	6	7
31. Informative	1	2	3	4	5	6	7
32. Humorous	1	2	3	4	5	6	7
33. Warm	1	2	3	4	5	6	7

Scoring Key for SSI

Attractive: Sum items 15, 16, 22, 23, 29, 30, 33;
                           divide by 7.

Interpersonally sensitive: Sum items 2, 5, 10, 11, 21, 25, 26, 28;
                           divide by 8.

Task oriented: Sum items 1, 3, 4, 7, 13, 14, 17, 18, 19, 20;
                           divide by 10

Filler items: 6, 8, 9, 12, 24, 27, 31, 32

RESOURCE G

Counseling Interview Rating Form

Counselor: <u>Lori Russell-Chapin</u>   Date: <u>6/2/04</u>

Observer: _____   Tape number: <u>1</u>

Observer: _____   Audio or video (please circle)

Supervisor: <u>A. Ivey</u>   Session Number: <u>2</u>

For each of the following specific criteria demonstrated, make a frequency marking every time the skill is demonstrated. Then assign points for consistent skill mastery using the ratings scales below. Active mastery of each skill receives a score of 2. Skills marked with an X should be seen consistently on every tape. List any observations, comments, strengths and weaknesses in the space provided. Providing actual counselor phrases is helpful when offering feedback.

Ivey Mastery Ratings

3 Teach the skill to clients (teaching mastery only)
2 Use the skill with specific impact on client (active mastery)
1 Use and/or identify the counseling skill (basic mastery)
  To receive an A on a tape, at least 52–58 points must be earned.
  To receive a B on a tape, at least 46–51 points must be earned.
  To receive a C on a tape, at least 41–45 points must be earned.

Specific Criteria		Frequency	Comments	Skill Mastery Rating
A. Opening/Developing Rapport				
1. Greeting	X	I	Stephen, it is good to see you again.	2
2. Role definition/ expectation				
3. Administrative tasks				
4. Beginning	X	I	What do you want to work on today?	2
B. Exploration phase/ defining the problem Microskills				
1. Empathy/rapport		I		2
2. Respect				2
3. Nonverbal matching	X			
4. Minimal encourager	X	I		

(continued)

RESOURCE G CONTINUED

Specific Criteria		Frequency	Comments	Skill Mastery Rating
5. Paraphrasing	X	I	So in order to be the man and maybe even take the place of your dad, you can't focus on your studies and fun thins like soccer because you have so much to do around the house	2
6. Pacing/leading	X	II	It is kind of boring in here.	2
7. Verbal tracking	X	I	Let's not talk then but read instead.	2
8. Reflect feeling	X	III	Stephen, that must have been so scary and sad when your dad died.	2
9. Reflect meaning	X	III	That must be a huge responsibility for the oldest man in your hours.	2
10. Clarifications				
11. Open-ended questions		III	Stephen, when was the last time you felt powerful and in control?	2
12. Summarization	X			
13. Behavioral description	X	I		
14. Appropriate closed question	X	IIII	Do you like to read?	2
15. Perception check	X			
16. Silence	X	IIII		2
17. Focusing	X	I		2
18. Feedback	X	I	You were very brave, Stephen.	2
C. Problem-Solving Skills/Defining Skills				
1. Definition of goals	X	I	Our goal is to work on your having more fun and studying harder.	2
2. Exploration/ understanding of concerns	X	II	What do you need to do to be have you contacted lately?"	
3. Development/ evaluation of alternatives	X	II		2
4. Implement alternative		I	So every time you place an X, you must come up with one idea how to have fun and study harder.	2
5. Special techniques		III	Let's play ball for awhile.	2
6. Process counseling				
D. Action Phase/ Confronting Incongruities				
1. Immediacy				
2. Self-disclosure		I	One of the last times I was devastated was when my dad died.	2
3. Confrontation				
4. Directives		IIIII	Tell me what things you have tried to make your hurt go away.	2
5. Logical consequences				
6. Interpretation				

Specific Criteria	Frequency	Comments	Skill Mastery Rating
E. Closing/Generalization			
1. Summarization of Content feeling	I	Your hurt was really big. You were able today to make it much smaller by talking about your thoughts and feelings. Would you like to borrow the book to read to Abe?	2
2. Review of plan	X I	What is one thing that you will work on and one thing that you will play?	2
3. Rescheduling	I	When shall we make the next appointment?	2
4. Termination of session			
5. Evaluation of session	X II	What will you take with you from our session today that you can use in the week to come?	2
6. Follow-up	X		
F. Professionalism			
1. Developmental level match	I		2
2. Ethics			
3. Professional (punctual, attire, etc.)			

G. Strengths

I liked the way you paced with Stephen. Your play therapy interventions worked well and assisted Stephen in talking.

Area(s) for Improvement

Next time be sure to explore Stephen's grief and attempts at grieving.

Total: 52

RESOURCE H

Name of Institution
Name of Program
Student Practicum/Internship Agreement

Directions

Please complete this form in duplicate, submit one copy to the university supervisor and retain one copy for your own personal student file.

- I have read and understand the (professional organization) ethical standards and will practice counseling in accordance with these standards. Any breach of these ethics or any unethical behaviors on my part will result in my removal from practicum/internship and a failing grade. Documentation of such behavior will become part of my permanent record.
- I agree to adhere to the administrative policies, rules, standards, and practices of the practicum/internship site, including the HIPAA regulations
- I understand that my responsibilities include keeping my practicum/internship supervisors and my university supervisor informed regarding my field experiences.
- I understand that I will not earn a passing grade in practicum/internship unless I demonstrate the specified minimal level of counseling skill, knowledge, and competence, and complete course requirements as mandated by my course instructor.
- I understand that I must show proof of liability insurance in the amount of at least $1,000,000/$3,000,000 to my university supervisor within 1 week of the semester or session start and before working with any clients. My insurance may come from any reputable malpractice agency.

Signature: _____

Date: _____

RESOURCE I

PRACTICUM/INTERNSHIP CONTRACT

This agreement is made on _____ by and between
                          (month/day/year)

_____
(Counseling Field Site)

and the Human Development Program at (institution). The agreement is
effective for a period from _____ to_____
                            (month/day/year)   (month/day/year)
for a minimum of 750 clock hours. Hours worked during University
holidays and breaks will be determined by the student and site based on
the needs of school or agency.

THE HUMAN DEVELOPMENT COUNSELING PROGRAM AGREES

1. to assign a University faculty liaison to facilitate communication between the University and the site.
2. to provide a profile of the student, an academic calendar, and a course syllabus for practicum/internship.
3. to notify the students that they must adhere to the administrative policies, rules, standards, schedules, and practices of the site.
4. that the faculty liaison shall be available for consultation with both site supervisors and students.
5. that the University supervisor is responsible for the assignment of a course grade.
6. that the student carries liability insurance in the amount of $1,000,000/$3,000,000 during the entire time this agreement is in effect.

THE PRACTICUM/INTERNSHIP SITE AGREES

1. to assign a practicum supervisor who has the appropriate credentials, time, and interest for training the student.
2. to provide opportunities for the student to engage in a variety of counseling activities under supervision and for evaluating the student's performance.
3. to provide the student with adequate work space, telephone, office supplies, and staff to conduct professional activities.
4. to provide supervisory contact, which involves some examination of student work using audio/video tapes and observation.
5. to provide written evaluation of student's work based on criteria established by the University Program.

(continued)

RESOURCE I CONTINUED

_____

   (Name)   (Address)   (Phone)   (SS#)
will be the primary-site supervisor. The training activities checked below
will be provided in sufficient amounts to allow an adequate evaluation of
the student's level of competence in each activity.

_____

   (Name)   (Phone)
will be the faculty liaison with whom the student and practicum site
supervisor will communicate regarding progress, problems, and
performance evaluation.

PRACTICUM/INTERNSHIP ACTIVITIES

_____ Individual Counseling   _____ Career Counseling
          personal/social/educational/
          occupational
_____ Group Counseling   _____ Supervision
          co-leading   individual
          leading   group
                                                  peer

_____ Intake Interviewing Conferences _____ Case
                                                  staff meeting
_____ Testing   _____ Psychoeducational
          administration   Activities parent
          analysis/interpretation   conferences
                                                  outreach programs
_____ Consultation   inservice

                                         _____ Multicultural
                                                  experiences

_____   _____
Site Supervisor   Date

RESOURCE J

Institution
Program of Study
LOG

WEEKLY TIME SCHEDULE   WEEK #
° = Direct Service Hours

Date	Location	Amount of Time°	Practicum/Internship Activity	Comments
_____	_____	_____	_____	_____
_____	_____	_____	_____	_____
_____	_____	_____	_____	_____
_____	_____	_____	_____	_____
_____	_____	_____	_____	_____
_____	_____	_____	_____	_____
_____	_____	_____	_____	_____
_____	_____	_____	_____	_____
_____	_____	_____	_____	_____
_____	_____	_____	_____	_____
_____	_____	_____	_____	_____
_____	_____	_____	_____	_____
_____	_____	_____	_____	_____

TOTALS:

This Week: **Semester:**

Total Hours: _____   Total Hours: _____

Direct Service Total: _____   Direct Service Total: _____

RESOURCE K

Client Informed Consent Form

I _____ agree
to be counseled by a practicum/intern student in the (*Program*) at (*Institution*). I further understand that I may participate in counseling interviews that will be audio taped, video taped, and/or viewed by practicum/intern students through the use of one-way observation windows. I understand that I will be counseled by a graduate student who has completed advanced course work in counseling. I understand that the student will be supervised by a faculty member of the (*Institution*) (*Program*) and an agency site supervisor.

Client's Signature: _____

Date of Birth: _____ Today's Date: _____

Counselor's Signature: _____

Effective Date: _____

Expiration Date: _____

RESOURCE L

Client Release Form

I agree for my child, _____, to be counseled during the (*date*) school year by _____, Counselor Intern in the (*Program*) at (*Institution*). I understand that my child may participate in counseling interviews that may be audio taped or video taped, and/or viewed by practicum/internship students through the use of one-way observation windows. I further understand that _____

_____ has completed advanced coursework in counseling/therapy and will counsel my child. I further understand that a (*Institution*) Professor and an on-site (*Institution*) supervisor will oversee the Counselor Intern.

_____ I agree for my child to be counseled by the Counselor Intern for the (*date*) school year and for those sessions to be video taped or audio taped.

_____ I agree for my child to be counseled by the Counselor Intern for the (*date*) school year; however, I do not wish for those sessions to be video taped or audio taped.

_____ I agree to have counseling information shared with: _____ Person(s)

Parent/Guardian Signature _____

Date _____

Student Signature _____

Counselor Intern Signature _____

Date _____

Date Effective _____ Date Contract Expires _____

RESOURCE M

SITE SUPERVISOR'S EVALUATION
OF STUDENT COUNSELOR'S PERFORMANCE

Suggested use: This form is to be used to evaluate overall performance in counseling. The form will be completed twice per term by the on-site supervisor. The form is appropriate for individual or group counseling.

Name of Student Counselor: _____

Name of Supervisor/Agency: _____

Date of Evaluation: _____

Period Covered by the Evaluation: _____

Directions: The supervisor is to circle the number which best evaluates student counselor performance in each category.

General Supervision Comments

	EXCEPTIONAL PERFORMANCE		REQUIRES ASSISTANCE		APPROPRIATE/ ACCEPTABLE PERFORMANCE	
1. Demonstrates a personal commitment in developing professional competencies.	1	2	3	4	5	6
2. Invests time and energy in becoming a counselor.	1	2	3	4	5	6
3. Accepts and uses constructive criticism to enhance self-development and counseling skills.	1	2	3	4	5	6
4. Engages in open, comfortable, and clear communication with peers and supervisors.	1	2	3	4	5	6
5. Recognizes own competencies and skills and shares these with peers and supervisors.	1	2	3	4	5	6
6. Recognizes own deficiencies and actively works to overcome them with peers and supervisors.	1	2	3	4	5	6
7. Completes case reports and records punctually and conscientiously.	1	2	3	4	5	6

The Counseling Process

8. Researches the referral prior to the first interview.	1	2	3	4		5	6
9. Keeps appointments on time.	1	2	3	4		5	6
10. Begins the interview smoothly.	1	2	3	4		5	6
11. Explains the nature and objectives of counseling when appropriate.	1	2	3	4		5	6
12. Is relaxed and comfortable in the interview.	1	2	3	4		5	6
13. Communicates interest in and acceptance of the client.	1	2	3	4		5	6
14. Facilitates client expression of concerns and feelings	1	2	3	4		5	6

General Supervision Comments

	EXCEPTIONAL PERFORMANCE		REQUIRES ASSISTANCE		APPROPRIATE/ ACCEPTABLE PERFORMANCE	
15. Focuses on the content of the client's problem.	1	2	3	4	5	6
16. Recognizes and resists manipulation by the client.	1	2	3	4	5	6
17. Recognizes and addresses positive affect of the client.	1	2	3	4	5	6
18. Recognizes and addresses negative affect of the client.	1	2	3	4	5	6
19. Is spontaneous in the interview.	1	2	3	4	5	6
20. Uses silence effectively in the interview.	1	2	3	4	5	6
21. Is aware of own feelings in the counseling session.	1	2	3	4	5	6
22. Communicates own feelings to the client when appropriate.	1	2	3	4	5	6
23. Recognizes and skillfully interprets the client's covert messages.	1	2	3	4	5	6
24. Facilitates realistic goal setting with the client.	1	2	3	4	5	6
25. Encourages appropriate action-step planning with the client.	1	2	3	4	5	6
26. Employs judgment in the timing and use of different techniques.	1	2	3	4	5	6

(continued)

27. Initiates periodic evaluation of goals,
    action-steps, and process during   1   2   3   4   5   6
    counseling.
28. Explains, administers, and interprets
    tests correctly.   1   2   3   4   5   6
29. Terminates the interview smoothly.   1   2   3   4   5   6

The Conceptualization Process

30. Focuses on specific behaviors and their
    consequences, implications,
    and contingencies.   1   2   3   4   5   6
31. Recognizes and pursues discrepancies
    and meaning of inconsistent information.   1   2   3   4   5   6
32. Uses relevant case data in planning *both*
    immediate and long-range goals.   1   2   3   4   5   6
33. Uses relevant case data in considering
    various strategies and their implication.   1   2   3   4   5   6
34. Bases decisions on a theoretically sound
    and consistent rationale of human behavior. 1   2   3   4   5   6
35. Is perceptive in evaluating the effects
    of own counseling techniques.   1   2   3   4   5   6
36. Demonstrates ethical behavior in the
    counseling activity and case management.   1   2   3   4   5   6

Additional Comments/Suggestions to Improve Performance

_____
_____
_____\
_____
_____
_____
_____

Date: _____ Signature of Supervisor:_____

My signature indicates that I have read the above report and have discussed the content with my site supervisor. It does not necessarily indicate that I agree with the report in part or in whole.

Date: _____ Signature of Student Counselor: _____

CONTINUING SELF-IMPROVEMENT: MAJOR SUPERVISION MODEL CATEGORIES

☞ *Supervision is a privilege and a must, especially when it is created with a trusted mentor.*

OVERVIEW

GOALS

KEY CONCEPTS: FINDING THE SUPERVISION MATCH FOR YOU

DEVELOPMENTAL MODELS OF SUPERVISION
PRACTICAL REFLECTION 1: DEVELOPMENTAL MODEL GROWTH AREAS

INTEGRATED MODELS OF SUPERVISION
PRACTICAL REFLECTION 2: ROLE AND FOCUS NEEDS

THEORY-SPECIFIC SUPERVISION MODELS
PRACTICAL REFLECTION 3: THEORETICAL ORIENTATION

A SUPERVISION VIDEOTAPING METHOD: INTERPERSONAL PROCESS RECALL
PRACTICAL REFLECTION 4: NEEDED IPR QUESTIONS

SUPERVISION AND THE CASE OF RACHEL
DEVELOPMENTAL SUPERVISION AND THE CASE OF RACHEL
INTEGRATED SUPERVISION AND THE CASE OF RACHEL
THEORETICALLY ORIENTED SUPERVISION AND THE CASE OF RACHEL
PRACTICAL REFLECTION 5: YOUR FAVORITE SUPERVISION MODEL
PRACTICAL REFLECTION 6: YOU AND YOUR SUPERVISION PERCEPTIONS

SUMMARY AND PERSONAL INTEGRATION
PRACTICAL REFLECTION 7: INTEGRATION

REFERENCES
RESOURCES N THROUGH O

OVERVIEW

Three conceptual models of supervision will be presented. In each model, the general skill of feedback is central, but the feedback process comes from an assumption underlying the basic tenets of the supervision models. This chapter begins by stressing the importance of relationship qualities between you, the student, and your supervisor. Throughout the chapter, you will have reflective opportunities to discover the supervision model that might best match your supervision needs, along with a supervisory method of viewing videotapes. Finally you will assess your supervision needs with a supervisee questionnaire.

GOALS

1. Understand three different categories of supervision models.
2. Examine how the Microcounseling Supervision Model relates to the different categories of supervision models.
3. Recognize how the Interpersonal Process Recall (IPR) Method can be utilized with most supervision models.
4. Apply the differing supervision models to the Case of Rachel.
5. Identify the supervision model(s) that best fit you and your counseling style and needs.

KEY CONCEPTS: FINDING THE SUPERVISION MATCH FOR YOU

Supervision: A distinctive manner of approach and response to a supervisee's needs.

As mentioned in Chapter 2, the Microcounseling Supervision Model (MSM) was introduced to you first as your foundation for learning the needed basic interviewing skills. There are many other supervision models that have emerged throughout the history of the helping professions. We offer additional models to help you as a student have a general understanding of the major categories of supervision: (1) developmental models, (2) integrated models, and (3) theoretical orientation–specific models.

Function: Major responsibilities in supervision of administration, education and support (Kadushin, 1992).

Much like studying your counseling theories, these supervision models have many similarities and differences. You will begin to notice that most supervision models emphasize the importance of a healthy supervisee and supervisor relationship, stress the importance of feedback and communication, and have a variety of supervisor tasks and functions. Holloway and Carrol (1999) suggest that it is the supervision tasks and roles plus their functions of those tasks that equal the supervision process.

Role: The supervisor role such as teacher, consultant, evaluator, and so on, depends on the needs of the supervisee/student.

In other words, if you combine the roles and responsibilities of the supervisor with your needs, the counselor in training, then you have a supervision process.

After those similarities, each model focuses on its essential and unique supervision tenets. As you read the following models, try to determine which model offers you what you need during your field experience. You might find that your attraction to different models depends on your differing supervision concerns with a variety of clients. The personal changes you experience as you learn and grow throughout your practicum and internship will also make a difference in your supervision needs! You may find that each model has something to offer you!

DEVELOPMENTAL MODELS OF SUPERVISION

The basic tenets formulating developmental models of supervision are that, as a student, you continue to grow at your own pace with differing needs and differing styles of learning. If this is true, then the major objective during developmental supervision is to discover your personal needs and focus on whatever it takes to maximize your strengths and minimize your liabilities.

Developmental stages: Supervisees progress through a series of predictable levels or stages as they learn the skills of the counseling process.

Personal style: Awareness of the natural preference and match assisting each counselor in discovering an approach to counseling and supervision.

To manage this developmental nature of learning, the manner in which you and your supervisor interact must also change. As you mature and grow, your needs and wants from your supervisors will also change. In individual counseling, we assess the developmental level of the client and choose a corresponding intervention. A parallel process occurs within developmental supervision.

For example, Stoltenberg (1981) and Stoltenberg and Delworth (1987) formulated a developmental supervision model describing distinct levels of supervisees: beginning, intermediate, advanced, and master counselor. During each level or stage, the job of the supervisor is to structure your supervision, moving from imitative and demonstrative functions at the beginning level to more competent and self-reliant functions at the advanced levels (McNeill, Stoltenberg & Delworth, 1992).

In this model, a strong emphasis is on better understanding you and others around you, your motivational levels, and your ability to become autonomous. Each level includes those three processes (awareness, motivation, and autonomy), and within each level are nine growth areas for you to focus. See Table 4.1 to better understand each level.

The nine growth areas are intervention, skill competence, assessment techniques, interpersonal assessment, client conceptualization, individual differences, theoretical orientation, treatment goals and plans, and professional ethics (Stoltenberg, McNeill & Delworth, 1998) In developmental

TABLE	**SUPERVISEE AND SUPERVISOR BEHAVIORS**	
	Supervisee	**Supervisor**
Beginning—Level 1	Little experience; dependent on the supervisor	Models needed skills and behaviors; teacher role
Intermediate—Level 2	Less imitative; strives for independence	Provides some structure but encourages exploration
Advanced—Level 3	More insightful and motivated; more autonomous sharing	Listens and offers suggestions when asked
Master Counselor—Level 4	Skilled interpersonally cognitively, and professionally	Provides collegial and consultative functions

Practical Reflection 1: Developmental Model Growth Areas

As you read about Stoltenberg and Delworth's Developmental Model, identify which level and growth area you currently reside. In which areas might you need and want to grow and learn more?

_____

_____

_____

_____

Focus: Specific growth areas for the student in training to concentrate including skill competence to personal awareness to interventions.

supervision, your job and your supervisor's job will be to help you to discover your strengths and locate your areas for improvement. Once you realize this strategy can be a life-long learning pattern, then you, as a helping professional, can be responsible for your own growth throughout your career.

INTEGRATED MODELS OF SUPERVISION

Often when helping professionals are asked about their theoretical orientation, many clinicians will state they are eclectic in their views. To assist those who favor eclecticism, integrated models of supervision were designed for those who work from multiple theoretical orientations. We have already presented our Microcounseling Supervision Model (MSM), which

---

Practical Reflection 2: Role and Focus Needs

What role and specific focus would you like your supervisor to display with each of your clients? Select a current case study and request what you need.

_____

_____

_____

_____

---

falls into the category of integrated supervision. It is our belief that MSM successfully combines and uses many of the skills from a variety of theories and supervision models.

Another example of integrated supervision is the Discrimination Model of Supervision. It has been widely researched and its supporters believe it is an inclusive approach to supervision; its roots are in technical eclecticism (Bernard & Goodyear, 1998). One of the main goals of the Discrimination Model of Supervision is to focus on your needs as a supervisee by being able to respond flexibly with any needed strategy, technique, and/or guidance.

It is situation specific, and your supervisor would emphasize two primary functions during each of your sessions: the supervisor's role and focus. There are three roles that your supervisor would take, based on your supervision needs: teacher, counselor, and consultant. You might require your supervisor to put on the teacher's hat and role and directly instruct and demonstrate constructs and skills. You might need your supervisor to be in the counselor's role to assist you in locating your "blind spots" or becoming aware of, perhaps, some personal countertransference issues. Finally, there may be times during supervision when you just need

Countertransference: Unresolved feelings that a helping professional unconsciously projects onto a client.

TABLE 4.2   AREAS OF FOCUS

Role Focus	Definition
Process	Examines how you communicate with your client.
Conceptualization	Explores your intentions behind the chosen skill interventions
Personalization	Identifies mannerisms used to interact with clients such as body language and voice intonation

your supervisor to bounce back and forth intervention ideas surrounding your client. Your supervisor becomes your colleague and consultant. Each of these roles emphasizes three areas of focus for skill-building purposes: process, conceptualization, and personalization. Study and review Table 4.2 for the definition of each focus areas.

THEORY-SPECIFIC SUPERVISION MODELS

Helping professionals who adhere to a specific school of thought and therapy (cognitive-behavioral, psychodynamic, Rogerian, and so on) may believe that naturally it is wise to supervise from that same theoretical orientation. The major advantage to you is that if you and your supervisor share the same theoretical orientation, it maximizes the modeling that can occur in supervision (Bernard & Goodyear, 1998). Your supervisor could demonstrate discipline-specific skills as well as integrate necessary theoretical constructs.

For example, if your supervisor follows a Rational Emotive Behavioral Therapy (REBT) theoretical orientation, then two main skills would be required during supervision. First you would need to identify the problem and irrational thinking of both you and your client. Then you and your supervisor would select ways to dispute and challenge those same irrational thoughts as a method for changing and learning new, productive thoughts and behaviors (Ellis, 1989; Woods & Ellis, 1996). Behavioral and cognitive behavioral supervisors will emphasize and expect you to demonstrate more technical mastery than most supervisors (Bernard & Goodyear, 1998). If your supervisor uses a person-centered approach, then the focus may be one of self discovery and awareness (Rogers, 1961).

Practical Reflection 3: Theoretical Orientation

Think of a supervision moment when your supervisor was demonstrating a specific theoretical orientation skill. For you, what would be the advantages of focusing on one theoretical orientation?

_____

_____

_____

_____

A Supervision Videotaping Method: Interpersonal Process Recall

We have presented three main supervisory models. Many models require that you videotape your counseling interviews or conduct your sessions in an actual live observation setting. One of the most widely used methods that your instructor may use in class is Kagan's Interpersonal Process Recall (IPR) (Haynes, Corey, & Moulton, 2003). Borders and Leddick (1988) conducted a national survey of counselor educators and found IPR to be one of two distinct methods used during supervision courses.

The main essence of IPR is to create a supervision environment where supervisees can safely analyze their communication styles and strategies. Kagan believes that most people act diplomatically and often do not say what they actually mean or feel. In supervision, then, your supervisor will encourage you to reflect and interpret your experience in the counseling session. (Kagan, 1980). The best way to do that is to view a videotape of a counseling session and simply stop the tape at any time to discuss essential personal and/or counseling issues.

It was the work of Norm Kagan and Allen Ivey that inspired the development of the Microcounseling Supervision Model that you practiced in Chapter 2. Using the Counselor Interview Rating Form (CIRF) while videotaping is an extension of Kagan's work. Study the following list to see the questions that could be asked while using the Interpersonal Process Recall method (Bernard & Goodyear, 1998, p. 102).

- What were your thoughts, feelings, and reactions? Did you want to express them at any time?
- What would you like to have said at this point?
- What was it like for you in your role as counselor?
- What thoughts were you having about the other person at that time?
- Had you any ideas about what you wanted to do with that?
- Were there any pictures, images, or memories flashing through your mind then?
- How do you imagine the client was reacting to you?
- How do you think the client was seeing you at this point?
- Did you sense that the client had any expectations of you at that point?
- What did you want to hear from the client?
- What message did you want to give the client? What prevented you from doing so?

Practical Reflection 4: Needed IPR Questions

If you could use the IPR supervision method of viewing videotaped sessions, which of the above questions would assist you the most during your supervision?

_____

_____

_____

_____

SUPERVISION AND THE CASE OF RACHEL

You have been studying the Case of Rachel throughout the first section of this book, integrating unique features of Rachel's case study. As we described different models of supervision, it may be helpful to imagine working with Rachel using the three supervision models offered. You read how we supervised Rachel using the initial Microcounseling Supervision Model. The main emphasis was on identifying and classifying essential interviewing counseling skills. Microcounseling Supervision fits into the category of Integrated Supervision, as any theoretical orientation could use this approach to supervision. Resource N, A Summary of Microcounseling Skills Used in Other Theories (Ivey & Ivey, 2003) provides a list of the theories using Microcounseling Supervision. As we offer examples using the three supervisory models described in this chapter, begin to formulate the supervision approach that best fits with you and your present needs.

Developmental Supervision and the Case of Rachel

You may need to review Rachel's case from previous chapters. She is an older woman whose husband recently died. Rachel's children were trying to help her cope but were interfering with her independence. In Chapter 2, the importance of case presentations is discussed. The actual narrative case presentation for the Case of Rachel is presented in Chapter 5. In that narrative report, Lori requested assistance on issues of effectiveness with self-disclosure, multi-axial diagnosis, Rachel's resistance, personal issues of death, focus of resources, and general strengths and liabilities.

If Dr. Ivey were supervising Lori, and he selected Stoltenberg's (1981) and Stoltenberg and Delworth's model of Developmental Supervision (1987), he would first assess Lori's level of functioning from Level 1 through 4. Dr. Ivey would need to look at Lori's awareness of self and others; her motivation toward the developmental process; and her independent thinking. From her supervision questions and general skills, Dr. Ivey may see Lori's functioning between Level 2 and 3 because she seems aware of her impact on Rachel. The focus of supervision may need to highlight client conceptualization and treat goals and plans. Dr. Ivey would gently encourage Lori to gain confidence in her own skill development.

Integrated Supervision and the Case of Rachel

You have already read Dr. Ivey's supervisory responses to Lori using the integrated Microcounseling Supervision Model. If Dr. Ivey were supervising Lori using the Discrimination Model of Supervision, what would he need to consider? First, he would have to decide which foci to select and which role to use to accomplish the needed supervision goal. Since this is the first session with Rachel and one of Lori's first clients, Dr. Ivey may choose to focus on Lori's basic intervention skills by being in the role of teacher and counselor. He may actually teach new skills and work on the Lori's effect on the client.

The elegance of Discrimination Supervision is that as Dr. Ivey continues to supervise Lori, his foci and roles change across and within sessions (Bernard & Goodyear, 1998). The cardinal rule of any integrative supervision is to customize supervision to meet the needs of the individual supervisee. In other words, "the 'how' of supervision should parallel the 'what' of supervision" (Norcross & Halgin, 1997, p. 210).

Theoretically Oriented Supervision and the Case of Rachel

If Dr. Ivey decided to supervise Lori using a psychotherapy theory-based supervision model, he would choose one theory adhering to it tenets throughout the supervisory process. Using cognitive-behavioral supervision, Dr. Ivey would focus on skills and strategies that Lori may want to use with Rachel. He may also challenge any irrational thoughts Lori may have about personal death issues and need for approval.

In Psychodynamic Supervision, additional emphasis may be on parallel process (Doehrmann, 1976). *Parallel process* is the dynamic that occurs in the client/therapist relationship that is played out in the supervisee/supervisor relationship. Dr. Ivey may focus on the resistance that Rachel had during the session and investigate what resistance Lori may have toward him.

Practical Reflection 5: Your Favorite Supervision Model

Review the models presented. Which one(s) best matches your counseling style and needs today?

_____

_____

_____

_____

Using supervision from Person-Centered Theory, Dr. Ivey would ensure that the basic facilitative conditions were in process throughout the supervision session. Dr. Ivey would emphasize unconditional positive regard, building trust, and creating a genuine environment for Lori to express self-doubts and fears about confidence in her counseling skills (Hackney & Goodyear, 1984).

You have now had the opportunity to read about several different supervision models. Take the time to discover more about you as a supervisee by taking the Supervisee Perception of Supervision (Olk & Friedlander, 1992). Answer the statements honestly as you take the inventory located in Resource O at the back of this chapter. Let your scores from the questionnaire assist you in further defining what you need from supervision.

Practical Reflection 6: You and Your Supervision Perceptions

Discuss what you learned from taking the Supervisee Perception of Supervision instrument. Which roles are in conflict and which seem unclear? Share your concerns with your colleagues and supervisor.

_____

_____

_____

_____

SUMMARY AND PERSONAL INTEGRATION

This chapter offered additional models of supervision for you to include in your supervisory knowledge base. Three categories of supervision models were presented:

- Developmental
- Integrated
- Theoretically oriented

Examples were offered for each category and your task was to determine which, if any, model was the best fit for your counseling style and needs. The IPR supervision method of viewing videotapes was offered. A Supervisee Perception of Supervision was offered to assist you in determining your supervisory needs and expectations.

Practical Reflection 7: Integration

As your supervision knowledge base increases, which Chapter 4 constructs will assist you the most in becoming a skilled helping professional? Explain.

_____

_____

_____

_____

REFERENCES

Bernard, J. M., & Goodyear, R.K. (1998). *Fundamentals of Clinical Supervision*. Needham Heights, MA: Allyn and Bacon.

Borders L.D. & Leddick G. R. (1988). A nationwide survey of supervisory training. Counseling Education and Supervision, 27(3), 271–283.

Doehrman, M. (1976). Parallel processes in supervision and psychotherapy. *Bulletin of the Menninger Clinic, 40*, 3–104.

Ellis, A. (1989). Thoughts on supervising counselors and therapists. *Psychology: A Journal of Human Behavior, 26*, 3–5.

Hackney, H. L., & Goodyear, R. K. (1984). Carl Rogers' client–centered supervision. In R. F. Levant & J. M. Schlep (Eds.). *Client-Centered Therapy and the Person-Centered Approach*. New York: Praeger.

Haynes, R., Corey, G., & Moulton, P. (2003). *Clinical Supervision in the Helping Professions: A Practical Guide*. Pacific Grove, CA: Brooks/Cole.

Holloway, E., & Carrol, M. (Eds.). (1999). *Training Counselling Supervisors: Strategies, Methods and Techniques*. London: Sage.

Ivey, A. E., & Ivey, M. B. (2003). *Intentional Interviewing and Counseling: Facilitating Client Development in a Multicultural Society*. (5th ed.). Pacific Grove, CA: Brooks/Cole.

Kadushin, A. (1992). *Supervision in Social Work* (3rd ed.). New York: Columbia University Press.

Kagan, N. (1980). Influencing human interaction—eighteen years with IPR. In A. K. Hess (Ed.). *Psychotherapy Supervision: Theory, Research and Practice* (pp. 262–86). New York: Wiley.

McNeil, B. W., Stoltenberg, C. D., & Romans, J. S. (1992). The integrated developmental model of supervision: Scale development and validation procedures. *Professional Psychology: Research & Practice 23*, 504–8.

Norcross, J. C., & Halgin, R. P. (1997). Integrative approaches to psychotherapy supervision. In J. C. E. Watkins (Ed.). *Handbook of Psychotherapy Supervision* (pp. 203–22). New York: Wiley.

Olk, M., & Frielander, M. L. (1992). Trainee's experiences of role conflict and role ambiguity in supervisory relationships. *Journal of Counseling Psychology, 39*, 389–97.

Rogers, C. R. (1961). *On Becoming a Person*. Boston: Houghton Mifflin.

Stoltenberg, C. D. (1981). Approaching supervision from a developmental perspective: The counselor-complexity model. *Journal of Counseling Psychology, 28*, 59–65.

Stoltenberg, C. D., & Delworth, U. (1987). *Supervising Counselors and Therapists*. San Francisco: Jossey-Bass.

Stoltenberg, C. D., McNeill, B. W., & Delworth, U. (1998). *IDM Supervision: An Integrated Developmental Model for Supervising Counselors and Therapists*. San Francisco: Jossey-Bass.

Woods, P. J., & Ellis, A. (1996). Supervision in rational emotive behavior therapy. *Journal of Rational-Emotive & Cognitive Behavior Therapy, 14*, 135–52.

MICROSKILL LEAD

Legend: ● = Frequent use of skill, ◐ = Common use of skill, ○ = Occasional use of skill

	Decisional counseling	Person centered	Behavioral (assertiveness training)	Solution oriented	Psychodynamic	Gestalt	Rational-emotive behavioral therapy	Feminist therapy	Business problem solving	Medical diagnostic interview	Traditional teaching	Student-centered teaching	Eclectic/metatheoretical
BASIC LISTENING SKILLS													
Open question	●	○	◐	●	◐	●	◐	●	◐	◐	◐	●	◐
Closed question	◐	○	●	◐	○	◐	◐	◐	◐	◐	●	◐	◐
Encourager	●	●	◐	◐	◐	◐	◐	◐	◐	○	◐	◐	◐
Paraphrase	●	●	◐	●	◐	○	◐	◐	◐	◐	○	●	◐
Reflection of feeling	●	●	◐	◐	◐	○	◐	◐	◐	◐	○	●	◐
Summarization	◐	◐	◐	●	◐	○	◐	◐	◐	◐	◐	●	◐
ADVANCED SKILLS													
Reflection of meaning	◐	●	○	○	◐	○	◐	○	○	○	○	◐	◐
Interpretation/reframe	◐	○	○	○	●	●	●	◐	◐	◐	○	◐	◐
Logical consequences	◐	○	◐	○	○	○	●	◐	●	◐	●	◐	◐
Self-disclosure	◐	●	○	○	○	◐	○	●	○	○	○	◐	◐
Feedback	◐	●	◐	◐	○	◐	●	◐	◐	○	○	●	◐
Advice/information/and others	◐	○	◐	○	○	◐	●	◐	●	●	●	●	◐
Directive	◐	○	●	○	○	●	●	◐	●	●	●	◐	◐
CONFRONTATION (Combined Skill)	◐	◐	◐	◐	◐	●	●	◐	◐	◐	◐	◐	◐
FOCUS													
Client	●	●	●	●	●	●	●	○	◐	◐	◐	●	◐
Main theme/problem	●	○	◐	●	◐	○	◐	◐	●	●	◐	●	◐
Other	◐	○	◐	◐	◐	◐	○	◐	○	○	○	◐	◐
Family	◐	○	◐	◐	◐	○	○	◐	○	○	○	○	◐
Mutuality	○	◐	○	◐	○	○	○	◐	○	○	○	◐	◐
Counselor/interviewer	○	◐	○	○	○	○	◐	◐	○	○	○	◐	◐
Cultural. environmental context	◐	○	◐	◐	○	○	○	●	◐	○	○	◐	◐
ISSUE OF MEANING (Topics, key words likely to be attended to and reinforced)	Problem solving	Relationship	Behavior problem solving	Problem solving	Unconscious motivation	Here and now behavior	Irrational ideas/logic	Problem as a "women's issue"	Problem solving	Diagnosis of illness	Information/factors	Student ideas/info./facts	Varies
AMOUNT OF INTERVIEWER TALK-TIME	Medium	Low	High	Medium	Low	High	High	Medium	High	High	High	Medium	Varies

LEGEND
● Frequent use of skill
◐ Common use of skill
○ Occasional use of skill

RESOURCE O

SUPERVISEE PERCEPTION OF SUPERVISION[*]

The following statements describe some problems that therapists in training may experience during the course of clinical supervision. Please read each statement and then rate the extent to which you have experienced difficulty in supervision in your most recent clinical training. I have experienced difficulty in my current or most recent supervision because:

	NOT AT ALL				VERY MUCH
1. I was not certain about what material to present to my supervisor.	1	2	3	4	5
2. I have felt that my supervisor was incompetent or less competent than I. I often felt as though I was supervising him or her.	1	2	3	4	5
3. I have wanted to challenge the appropriateness of my supervisor's recommendations for using a technique with one of my clients, but I have thought it better to keep my opinions to myself.	1	2	3	4	5
4. I wasn't sure how best to use supervision as I became more experienced, although I was aware that I was undecided about whether to confront my supervisor.	1	2	3	4	5
5. I have believed that my supervisor's behavior in one or more situations was unethical or illegal and I was undecided about whether to confront him or her.	1	2	3	4	5
6. My orientation to therapy was different from that of my supervisor. She or he wanted me to work with clients using her or his framework, and I felt that I should be allowed to use my own approach.	1	2	3	4	5
7. I have wanted to intervene with one of my clients in a particular way and my supervisor has wanted me to approach the client in a very different way. I am expected both to judge what is appropriate for myself and also to do what I am told.	1	2	3	4	5
8. My supervisor expected me to come prepared for supervision, but I had no idea what or how to prepare.	1	2	3	4	5

[*]Olk, M. & Friedlander, M.L. (1992). Trainee's experiences of role conflict and role ambiguity in supervisory relationships. Journel of Psychology, 39, 389–397. Copyright © 1992 by the American Psychological Association. Reprinted (or Adapted) with permission.

	NOT AT ALL				VERY MUCH SO

9. I wasn't sure how autonomous I should be in my
   work with clients.   1   2   3   4   5
10. My supervisor told me to do something I perceived
    to be illegal or unethical and I was expected to comply.   1   2   3   4   5
11. My supervisor's criteria for evaluating my work
    were not specific.   1   2   3   4   5
12. I was not sure that I had done what the supervisor
    expected me to do in a session with a client.   1   2   3   4   5
13. The criteria for evaluating my performance in
    supervision were not clear.   1   2   3   4   5
14. I got mixed signals from my supervisor and I was
    unsure of which signals to attend to.   1   2   3   4   5
15. When using a new technique, I was unclear about the
    specific steps involved. As a result I wasn't sure how
    my supervisor would evaluate my work.   1   2   3   4   5
16. I disagreed with my supervisor about how to introduce
    a specific issue to a client, but I also wanted to do what
    the supervisor recommended.   1   2   3   4   5
17. Part of me wanted to rely on my own instincts with
    clients, but I always knew that my supervisor
    would have the last word.   1   2   3   4   5
18. The feedback I got from my supervisor did not
    help me to know what was expected of me in my day
    to day work with clients.   1   2   3   4   5
19. I was not comfortable using a technique recommended
    by my supervisor; however, I felt that I should do what
    my supervisor recommended.   1   2   3   4   5
20. Everything was new and I wasn't sure what would
    be expected of me.   1   2   3   4   5
21. I was not sure if I should discuss my professional
    weaknesses in supervision because I was not sure how
    I would be evaluated.   1   2   3   4   5
22. I disagreed with my supervisor about implementing
    a specific technique, but I also wanted to do what the
    supervisor thought best.   1   2   3   4   5
23. My supervisor gave me no feedback and I felt lost.   1   2   3   4   5
24. My supervisor told me what to do with a client,
    but didn't give me very specific ideas about how to do it. 1   2   3   4   5

(continued)

RESOURCE O CONTINUED

	NOT AT ALL				VERY MUCH SO
25. My supervisor wanted me to pursue an assessment technique that I considered inappropriate for a particular client.	1	2	3	4	5
26. There were no clear guidelines for my behavior in supervision.	1	2	3	4	5
27. The supervisor gave no constructive or negative feedback and as a result I did not know how to address my weaknesses.	1	2	3	4	5
28. I didn't know how I was doing as a therapist and as a result I didn't know how my supervisor would evaluate me.	1	2	3	4	5
29. I was unsure of what to expect from my supervisor.	1	2	3	4	5

Scoring Key

Role ambiguity items: 1, 4, 8, 9, 11, 12, 13, 18, 20, 21, 23, 24, 26, 27, 28, 29
Role conflict items: 2, 3, 5, 6, 7, 10, 14, 15, 16, 17, 19, 22, 25

Meaning

Look at the responses for each statement. High scores of 4's and 5's validate your feelings and beliefs concerning role ambiguity and role conflict. These concerns need to be shared in supervision.

CONCEPTUALIZING THE CLIENT: DIAGNOSIS AND RELATED ISSUES

🖙 *Multiaxial diagnosing is like discovering five more pieces to the conceptualization and treatment puzzle.*

OVERVIEW

GOALS

KEY CONCEPTS: CLIENT CASE CONCEPTUALIZATION AND THE INVESTIGATIVE NATURE OF COUNSELING
CONFIDENTIALITY
HUMBLE GUEST
CAUTIOUSNESS

CASE CONCEPTUALIZATION METHODS
USING THE INTERVIEW STAGES TO CONCEPTUALIZE CASES
PRACTICAL REFLECTION 1: STAGES OF THE INTERVIEW
ADDING THE DSM-IV-TR TO THE CASE CONCEPTUALIZATION

DIAGNOSIS USING THE DSM-IV-TR
DSM-IV-TR AXIS I—CLINICAL SYNDROMES AND OTHER CONDITIONS THAT MAY BE A FOCUS OF CLINICAL ATTENTION
DSM-IV-TR AXIS II—PERSONALITY DISORDERS AND MENTAL RETARDATION
DSM-IV-TR AXIS III—GENERAL MEDICAL CONCERNS
DSM-IV-TR AXIS IV—PSYCHOSOCIAL AND ENVIRONMENTAL PROBLEMS
DSM-IV-TR AXIS V—GLOBAL ASSESSMENT OF FUNCTIONING

PRACTICAL REFLECTION 2: DSM-IV-TR STRATEGY AND CONCEPTUALIZATION

DEVELOPMENTAL ASSESSMENT
PRACTICAL REFLECTION 3: YOUR PREFERRED DEVELOPMENTAL ORIENTATION

GOALS AND TREATMENT PLANS
CASE PRESENTATION GUIDELINES
NARRATIVE CASE PRESENTATION ABOUT RACHEL
PRACTICAL REFLECTION 4: CASE PRESENTATION ADDITIONS

THE CASE OF RACHEL: CASE CONCEPTUALIZATION WITH THE STAGES OF THE INTERVIEW, CLINICAL DIAGNOSIS, AND DEVELOPMENTAL ASSESSMENT
STAGES OF THE INTERVIEW
DSM-IV-TR DIAGNOSIS
DEVELOPMENTAL ASSESSMENT
GOALS AND TREATMENT FOR RACHEL

SUMMARY AND PERSONAL INTEGRATION
PRACTICAL REFLECTION 5: INTEGRATION

REFERENCES
RESOURCES P THROUGH Q

OVERVIEW

The purpose of this chapter is to introduce you to the world of case conceptualization and how it relates to formal client diagnostic systems such as the American Psychiatric Association's *Diagnostic and Statistical Manual of Mental Disorders, Text Revision*, 4th edition (DSM-IV-TR) (APA, 2000). There are many variables involved in the conceptualization and understanding of your client's world. In this chapter, you will be introduced to three case conceptualization strategies: Stages of the Counseling Interview, DSM-IV-TR, and Developmental Assessment. These strategies can be used independently and stand alone as methods of conceptualizing your cases. However, these approaches also work well together to provide you with an in-depth and comprehensive view of your client's world. You will utilize the stages of the counseling interview to provide structure to your conceptualization, dissect each of the five DSM-IV-TR axes used in multi-axis diagnosing, and view diagnosis from a developmental perspective. At the end of this chapter, you will delve into conceptualization using the Case of Rachel.

GOALS

1. Identify some key issues involved in client case conceptualization.
2. Work with three case conceptualization strategies.
3. Understand how the stages of the counseling interview provide a framework for conceptualizing your cases.
4. Focus on the five axes of the *Diagnostic and Statistical Manual of Mental Disorders–IV–Text Revision* (DSM-IV-TR) and how they relate to conceptualization, regardless of placement setting.
5. Understand how developmental assessment assists in treatment interventions.
6. Use case conceptualization and diagnosis as a tool for enhancing effective counseling and treatment with the Case of Rachel.

KEY CONCEPTS: CLIENT CASE CONCEPTUALIZATION AND THE INVESTIGATIVE NATURE OF COUNSELING

The world of case conceptualization and its relationship to formal client diagnostic systems such as the DSM-IV-TR (APA, 2000) is a fascinating and essential aspect of counseling. Client case conceptualization is like

Diagnostic and Statistical Manual for Mental Disorders, Fourth Edition, Text Revision (DSM-IV-TR): A text revision of the fourth edition of a classification manual published by the American Psychiatric Association coding over 400 different classifications.

Diagnosis: The use of an assessment tool or strategy to analyze a person's functioning and symptomatology.

being a detective in a mystery case. Each new piece of information tells a different and unique aspect of this major problem that your client has allowed you to hear, see, and investigate. Often once you have put the puzzle pieces together, you may finally see the gestalt of the problem.

Whether you choose to include active diagnosis of your clients as a part of client case conceptualization is a decision you must make with your on-site supervisor and university instructor. Regardless of your diagnosis position, it is essential that you be familiar with the diagnostic process to read the diagnoses of other professionals in the helping professions. Diagnosis can serve as common and universal communication tools, bringing together clinicians working with people's social, emotional, and physiologic concerns.

Your major task is, of course, to work on understanding the client and helping that client achieve counseling goals and resolve issues. Multiaxial diagnosis may offer additional information about the client and case conceptualization. You may use the diagnostic process as yet another piece of information to the puzzle of effective treatment.

Conceptualizing a client's case can be a stimulating and interesting journey. It is a journey that you must not take alone, because it is your client's world and perspective and also includes your supervisor's perspective. If you allow your client and supervisor to be active players of the case conceptualization and treatment team, the three of you can learn together. With this team approach, counseling gains and outcomes are more realistic, practical, and efficient.

As you join with your client in asking the needed questions and working together as team players, three cautionary statements must be mentioned.

Confidentiality

The world of counseling builds therapeutic relationships like none other. Often people enter your life when they are the most vulnerable, afraid, and fragile. One of the reasons the process of counseling works is that you, as the counselor, demonstrate to the client that this place of sharing and working is a safe haven. Your client must know that all material shared is confidential, unless you believe the client may be harmful to self or others. As you know, it is this confidentiality that many times is the reason people enter into the frightening journey of self-awareness and growth. Be sure you demonstrate confidentiality by your words, attitudes, and consistent behaviors.

Humble Guest

Another variable that helps in case conceptualization, diagnosing, and treatment is the attitude of respect that you emanate to your client. You have been invited into your client's life as a humble guest. It is a place of honor at the head table. If you have never been in personal counseling as a client, consider your field experience as an opportunity to get into counseling. There are two reasons for seeking counseling yourself. Remember that you can only take your clients as far as you have gone yourself! You need to be as healthy as possible to serve your clientele. Even more importantly, though, you must know what it is like to have the courage to ask a stranger for assistance! Lori has been in counseling three times throughout her life history. The first time was in her doctoral program, when everyone was gently encouraged to enter into counseling. She went begrudgingly, feeling invaded and resentful! Lori also felt scared, embarrassed, and finally relieved, and the list goes on. Allen did years of psychoanalytically oriented therapy and found it extremely beneficial in terms of self-learning and growth. Both of us believe that it assisted us in terms of a broader understanding of what is going on with our clients!

From those first counseling experiences, you will learn to surrender to your fears and ask for help. From your position as a client, you will learn how to gain needed strength and new coping skills. Everyone has problems, no one is exempt, and everyone can benefit from a respectful, counseling relationship, *if* you, as the counselor, understand your position of humbled guest. There is no greater honor than being asked to be a part of someone's life who is struggling and scared. No trust has even been established when that client walks into your office. It is your first counseling task to honor that client, no matter where they are in life, and begin the delicate task of creating a trusting counseling relationship! You can accomplish that by meeting the client wherever they are and conscientiously beginning to gather all the needed information for case conceptualization, diagnosis, and treatment.

Cautiousness

There are many levels of case conceptualization that will be developed throughout the chapter; however, when it comes to case conceptualization and diagnosing using the DSM-IV-TR, it is a serious matter. Once you have gathered all your needed information, formally checked the criteria in the DSM-IV-TR, and discussed the aspects of the case with your supervisor, you are finally ready to apply a diagnosis to the five axes. Please remember that your work and diagnosis may travel with the client wherever he or she goes.

If you choose to use diagnosis as part of your case conceptualization, remember that many people may view your diagnosis, such as other involved helping professionals, insurance companies, and possibly your client. Your client does have the right to view his personal file, and many clients find it helpful if they are part of the naming process that is diagnosis. Consider encouraging your client to be an active participant.

A DSM diagnosis is a serious label and must be accomplished through diligent work and knowledge. As with all aspects of your counseling job, take this part of your job very seriously and be cautious with your attitudes about quickly and nonchalantly writing down symptoms, diagnoses, and treatment goals.

CASE CONCEPTUALIZATION METHODS

There are many methods available for viewing the client's worldview and strategically assessing and intervening on the problem. One client conceptualization method that has already been presented to you utilizes the same interview stages presented in the Microcounseling Supervision Model: rapport/structuring, defining the problem, defining the goal, exploration of alternatives, and generalization to daily life (Ivey & Ivey, 2003). You can review those stages in Resource C and by using the Counseling Interview Rating Form (CIRF).

Using the Interview Stages to Conceptualize Cases

It is essential that you be able to understand the basics of case conceptualization; how you view your client's world and concerns certainly influences your treatment of that client. Using the stages of the interview to assist you in building your case is a natural approach to case conceptualization. Please take a look at the CIRF or view the Microskills Hierarchy in Resource P. Follow along as we describe each stage.

Notice in the first two stages—rapport building/structuring and exploration/defining the problem—that many of the essential interviewing skills are used. The intention behind all of these basic skills is to encourage your client to share the concerns that are a focus of the counseling interview. It is at this point that you encourage your client to "tell the story." This is the very first phase of the client's case conceptualization.

The most fundamental issue in conceptualization is, what is going on with the client? What are her or his concerns? What might have brought about the problem? What are some critical systems that might impact the client (family, work, and so on)? It is during these two stages that you may begin to use the diagnostic approach to case conceptualization.

During the third stage of the interview, defining goals and problem solving, your task is to analyze the information gleaned and set appropriate goals. What are the counseling goals? The fourth stage, action and confronting incongruities, is very dynamic and fluid. As client progress is

---

Practical Reflection 1: Stages of the Interview

How will the stages of the counseling interview assist you in conceptualizing your cases? Use the stages of the counseling interview to conceptualize a current client's case.

_____

_____

_____

_____

---

achieved and new awarenesses are gained, you can continue to set new goals and action strategies.

The final stage of closing and generalization assists in case conceptualization by tying up loose ends, summarizing outcomes, and evaluating present and future needs. The stages work together providing you with seamless clues that create a final but ever-growing case agenda. You can use these five stages as a way to organize your interviewing notes, plus you can use this model to summarize and conceptualize the interview. You can use it for notes and long-term treatment planning.

A similar conceptualization method is the three-stage Skilled Helper Model (Egan, 2002) delineating Stage 1, What's going on?; Stage II, What solution makes sense for me?; and Stage III, How do I get what I need or want? It is your responsibility as the helping professional to understand the issues and conceptualize the solutions, regardless of the method you choose.

Adding the DSM-IV-TR to the Case Conceptualization

As you develop and conceptualize each case, remember whether you decide to follow the Diagnostic and Statistical Manual, Fourth Edition and Text Revision (DSM-IV-TR) multiaxial approach or not is a decision you must make. If you find it helpful to do so, then diagnose on all five axes. If making a diagnosis on axis I or II is more helpful, then follow that strategy. You must follow your agency guidelines as well, but each decision on using the multiaxial approach can be determined on a client to client basis.

In the past, many counselor educators and social workers believed that there was no place for diagnosing in counseling. Interviewers, more often than not, assist people in effectively dealing with everyday problems and life issues. Counselors main charge is prevention, not labeling clients as mentally ill (Kjos, 1994). However, as the counseling and social work field became more receptive to the idea of clinical diagnosis, the definition of diagnosis expanded to include different aspects and layers. Although we still work with everyday life problems, the prevalent thinking is that all clinicians working in the helping professions must understand the dynamics of the major classification systems to more effectively work with each other.

DIAGNOSIS USING THE DSM-IV-TR

The DSM-IV-TR provides a guideline allowing you to investigate your client's concerns using a multiaxial approach. Diagnosing on the five DSM-IV-TR axes provides you with the opportunity to view your client's world in a much broader manner. All helping professions need to understand and familiarize themselves with the DSM-IV-TR to competently serve their clientele (Kjos, 1994).

DSM-IV-TR Axis I—Clinical Syndromes and Other Conditions That May Be a Focus of Clinical Attention

Axis I is the first piece of the clinical diagnosis and comes in the form of the presenting problem(s) or major focus of clinical attention. You gather this information from the Client Intake Form, the client's own words, and your initial observations after the first intake interview. You can certainly create your own intake form, but please remember to use the forms from your university and field experience agencies and schools first.

Often students ask what they should do if their opinions and observations are different from what the client says is the presenting problem. If the client says the presenting problem is a marriage concern, but during your interview, you obtained material that may suggest your client is also alcoholic, there seems to be a conflict about what the focus should be. Your client is telling you the reason she came into counseling is her failing marriage, but you suspect a deeper and separate issue.

There are two different strategies you can follow. First, in a purely ethical sense, it seems logical to write down the presenting problem that your client states is the problem and is currently willing to admit. As the counselor, you can now offer a dual diagnosis using both labels, providing both situations fit. You can also provide a "rule out" as an option, demonstrating that your client may fit this category, but you are not certain and must perform more assessments and obtain more quantitative evidence to rule out this possibility. With this example, it is very difficult to focus on a troubled marriage, if your client is dealing with alcoholism concerns.

Clients are not generally willing to tell you exactly what the counseling problem is because it is too scary, too embarrassing, and/or too unknown. Once trust has been established, you can ask an essential exploratory question, "What do you need to tell me that you have been keeping to yourself?" This level of trust allows you to finally get to the depth of the issues. Bergman (1985) refers to this as "fishing for the barracuda!" This part of your investigation is critical to your diagnosis for axes I and II, and it is the underlying essence of effective diagnosis and treatment. Until clients feel comfortable enough to trust you with the secrets that they have been hiding for many years, you may not discover that flesh-eating barracuda. Once you find it, you can always change your axis I diagnosis and your focus of clinical attention. For the most part, however, your axis I diagnosis needs to be the client's perceptions of the problem and clinical syndromes and symptoms presented.

Here are the three basic questions you need to be able to answer when diagnosing on axis I: (1) What are the major psychiatric symptoms and disorders? (2) What developmental issues are arrested or are currently presenting difficulty? (3) What is their duration and how does their intensity vary (Ginter, 2002)? These questions integrate well with the questions you asked in stages I and II of the interview. Hopefully, you are beginning to see how using the interview stages and the DSM-IV-TR can work together.

DSM-IV-TR Axis II—Personality Disorders and Mental Retardation

Personality disorders: An axis II classification describing severe personality dysfunctioning that causes disturbances in thinking and actions on a daily basis.

Axis II is the second piece of the clinical diagnosis and addresses personality disorders and mental retardation. Both of these classifications must be objectively and quantifiably measured to ensure the accuracy of the problem. Many clinicians use the DSM-IV Manual and its criteria to indicate severe pathologies. This is a useful method for corroborating your appraisal results, but please never use the criteria alone. It is best to always defer your personality disorder labels using the code of 799.9 (deferred diagnosis code for axis I and II) until you can actually test your client for personality disorders and mental retardation.

There are many valid and reliable instruments assessing these conditions. Two of the best personality instruments are the Millon Clinical Multiaxial Inventory (MCMI) (Millon, 1994) and the Minnesota Multiphasic Personality Instrument (MMPI) (Hathaway & McKinley, 1989). Both tests can be scored by hand or computer; however, the hand-scoreable tests offer a more individualized profile because the results refer to only your client. When using a computerized form, the profile is individualized but the treatment suggestions are generic and compared to others having a similar profile. The results are immediate, however. Be cautious and experienced using these tests. When sharing information with clients regarding the results, we do not recommend that you or your supervisor share actual test scores. Remember that your client's life does depend on accurate diagnosis. If a score must be reported, try sharing the standard error of measurement as the central concept.

The two best protocols for assessing mental retardation are the Weschler scales from early childhood on to adults and the Standford-Binet test. These instruments have been thoroughly researched for validity and reliability, and like the personality tests, are widely utilized in assessing client needs.

Determining and objectively analyzing personality disorders are critical steps in the treatment of your client. If your client does score in the personality disorder range, you understand the intensity of your client's concern. A personality disorder influences and affects your client's decision making on a daily basis. The sooner the client understands the impact of the disorder, the more quickly you can assist him or her in becoming more aware of those needs.

Here are the essential questions you need to ask for determining the diagnosis for axis II: (1) Are there any lifelong maladaptive patterns or traits? (2) Do these patterns tend to cause trouble in intimate, social, or work relationships (Ginter, 2002)? Again, these questions fit nicely into Stage II, defining the problem.

DSM-IV-TR Axis III—General Medical Concerns

Another piece of the clinical puzzle is offered through the axis III diagnosis. This axis provides information about medical concerns and conditions that affect axis I assessment. For example, if your axis I diagnosis is alcohol dependence and your client is also found to have cirrhosis of the liver, then one of your first goals is to ensure that the liver issues are being addressed. Once physiologic needs are leveled out, cognitive and socioemotional concerns can more effectively be addressed.

International Classifications of Diseases (ICD-10): Another manual coding medical and psychiatric disorders published through the World Health Organization.

Axis III medical concerns are coded using the International Classification of Diseases (ICD-10) numbers in the DMS-IV-TR. This section is categorized into medical sections, such as *Diseases of the Nervous System, Diseases of the Circulatory System, Diseases of the Respiratory System, Endocrine Diseases, Nutritional Diseases, Metabolic Diseases, Digestive System Diseases, Genitourinary Diseases, Hematological Diseases of the*

Eye, Ear, Nose and Throat, Musculoskeletal Diseases, Skin Diseases, Congenital Diseases, Diseases of Pregnancy and Childbirth, and *Infectious Diseases* (APA, 2000).

Please remember to code only those medical concerns that are related to your axis I diagnosis. The essential questions you need to address in diagnosing in axis III are twofold: (1) Are there medical problems that need to be considered? (2) How do they affect psychiatric symptoms and potential treatment planning (Ginter, 2002)? These questions aid your discovery process during Stages I and II of the interview.

DSM-IV-TR Axis IV—Psychosocial and Environmental Problems

Psychosocial stressors: Any environmental and social concerns that may influence the focus of clinical attention in axis I is indicated on axis IV.

An important aspect of understanding and treating your client is to recognize the additional variables and psychosocial stressors that contribute to the client's problems. These variables may not be the main clinical focus of your attention, but the role these extra conditions play may be instrumental to the wellness and treatment of your client. If the client who is alcohol dependent and has cirrhosis of the liver also is struggling in her marriage and may lose her job, then all these stressors affect your treatment plans. These additional stressors are listed on axis IV in narrative form. The descriptions of many of the variables are listed in the DSM-IV-TR as V codes. Ginter (2002) suggests that two questions must be answered for axis IV diagnosis: (1) What psychosocial or environmental problems need to be addressed? (2) How effective is the client's coping repertoire? These questions address and supplement situational and developmental concerns that you are seeking in Stages I and II of the interview.

DSM-IV-TR Axis V—Global Assessment of Functioning

Global Assessment of Functioning (GAF): An axis V coding system from 0 to 100 for assessing the level of symptomatology of a client; 0 shows suicidal actions and thoughts and 100 shows no present symptomatology.

The final axis is another clue to your clients' overall developmental functioning. The DSM-IV-TR manual lists the intensity and corresponding symptomatology on a rating scale from 0 to 100 (APA, 2000). For example, in the Global Assessment of Functioning (GAF) continuum of 1 to 10, the description reads, "Persistent danger of severely hurting self or others (e.g., recurrent violence) or persistent inability to maintain minimal personal hygiene or serious suicidal act with clear expectation of death" (APA, 1994, p. 47). Compare that to the range of 81 to 90, "Absent or minimal symptoms (e.g. mild anxiety before an exam), good functioning in all areas, interested and involved in a wide range of activities, socially effective, generally satisfied with life, no more than everyday problems or concerns (e.g., an occasional argument with family members) (APA, 1994, p. 46).

Practical Reflection 2: DSM-IV-TR Strategy and Conceptualization

List your major concerns about diagnosing using the DSM-IV-TR multiaxial approach. Which axes will offer you the most helpful information for conceptualizing your case?

_____

_____

_____

_____

Although you are the helping professional selecting the rating, it is based on subjective and objective data. As a beginning counselor, you also need to realize that diagnosis is often subjective. If five expert clinicians were asked to diagnosis the very same case, there well could be five very different assessments, indications, and coding diagnosis. Don't let this alarm you; each clinician has a different expertise and different perceptions about the case in question. There would be some similarities between the codes, but the treatment focus may be seen through a unique set of occupational filters. There are four questions that need to be answered before your axis V diagnosis can be complete: (1) What kind of resources can the individual bring to bear (personal, social, and so on)? (2) How well are they functioning socially and in their intimate relationships? (3) How well are they functioning academically? (4) What can you expect in terms of their overall prognosis (Ginter, 2002)?

DEVELOPMENTAL ASSESSMENT

Developmental assessment: Matching the counseling language style with the client's organizational reference to the world.

The third and final strategy adding to your case conceptualization is developmental assessment. As you have learned, stages of the interview and clinical diagnosis offer information about the client's problems, but development diagnosis offers information about your client's style and orientation to the world. Proponents of assessing the developmental levels (Ashen, 1977; Ivey & Ivey, 1998) emphasize that clients enter into the counseling system from an individual and familiar cognitive and emotional frame of reference. Even the authors of the DSM-IV-TR are beginning to recognize how development and culture may interface with diagnostic concerns. Smart and Smart (1997) researched DSM-IV changes and concluded that 79 out of 400 disorders now address some cultural descriptions.

Ivey and Ivey (2003) suggest that clients offer you clues about how their world is arranged and organized. By matching your words and phrases with the client's worldview, you build rapport and let the client know you do understand the presented views. There are four developmental levels discussed and four recommended appropriate intervention types to match these levels. Your counseling task is to listen and observe very carefully and match the client's beginning developmental orientation with similar skills and theories. Once that is accomplished, you can intentionally mismatch to assist the client in developmental stretching.

Developmental style 1 (D-1) is a sensorimotor orientation. A client in this style feels and shows emotion deeply and may feel overwhelmed and in a state of crisis. An appropriate development response may be to listen and then respond with a structured directive, assisting the client to move in a positive direction.

We will use a hypothetical Susie as an example. Assume that Susie is seeking you to talk about mild, but possibly clinical depression. Susie's example statement: Susie begins to weep, "I can't believe my husband is so mean to me and the kids. I am crushed." Her presentation of her problems is somewhat random and it is hard to follow her logic. She is deeply embedded in her emotions.

Clients in the developmental style 2 (D-2) are in the concrete orientation style. These clients are often linear and detailed. Their account of the situation is specific, and the stories are long and involved. In this style, Susie's example statement is: "This morning I woke up at 5:30. I cleaned the house and fed the dog. I got the kids up and dressed at 7:00, had breakfast, and we made the beds. As we were leaving the house, my husband became very critical about the mail piling up and how lazy we all were. We all left the house in tears."

You will find that many clients present their issues in this fashion, and it is important to listen carefully and not become bored or to push the client to reflection and analysis too soon. Paraphrasing and summarization can be especially helpful because it shows the client that they have been heard; they many not need to repeat their stories several times.

A developmental style of formal-operational orientation (D-3) is demonstrated with little detail and feelings, but your client may talk in abstract terms about the problem. Themes, patterns, and self-analysis seem to come easily to people in this style. Susie's example statement: "It tends to always be the same. I try so hard to please him and be a good wife and mother. Perhaps that is the problem, I am trying too hard, but whenever

I try hard, my husband becomes critical and harsh." Here you see a more verbal client, one who is often good at examining the self and patterns of thought, action, and feeling.

The final developmental style is dialectic/systemic orientation (D-4). A client in this style tends to have a need to analyze patterns with self but also the contextual situation. Susie's example statement: "Probably there are many ways to look at this problem. I am sure that when I am overwhelmed and trying hard to keep everything and everybody together and happy, that there must be that stress spillover to everyone around me."

This brief discussion of developmental assessment can be valuable to you in several ways. First, it reminds you that clients present their issues in varying styles and that it is essential to meet the client where he or she is at the moment. As clients progress and change, you will find that their verbal style changes, and you will want to change your mode of working with them. This strategy of developmental assessment has specific implications for treatment as well.

Ashen (1977) offers another method for developmental assessment. He believes that all people carry mental pictures in their minds of certain situations. It is not until these symbols or images become conscious that the client will be able to make direct and rational choices about these events. A triadic model is presented, demonstrating that clients enter the counseling system using created images (I), somatic responses (S), and related meaning (M). Whichever component a client chooses, is the one you want to use. Once the client knows you understand him or her, then it is the counselor's job to gently stretch the client for further understanding of the problem.

For example, a client enters counseling stating he is very sad, depressed, and he does not feel productive at work. Your client has offered the meaning (M) component of the triad. It is your job to hook into that meaning component by understanding all of its dimensions, then gently begin to stretch to the other components looking for additional clues to fill in the treatment story. What are the somatic and physiologic symptoms? If he has headaches, when and where does your client most often develop these headaches? What are these headaches telling him from a symbolic point of view? This last question may lead you into the image component of the triad by listening to your client's wordings and phrasings: His headaches might be stating that he feels like he is between a rock and a hard place. You need to carefully examine his images of "a rock and a hard place."

These developmental assessments offer another strategy in the diagnosis and treatment aspects of counseling. When you imagine the advantages of developmental assessments and combine those clues offered with the counseling stages and clinical diagnosis, your counseling puzzle is

Practical Reflection 3: Your Preferred Developmental Orientation Style

Think back to a time in your life when you were describing one of your problems to a friend or helping professional. Did you offer feelings, thoughts, details, images? What developmental orientations (D-1 through D-4) did you present? Sensorimotor? Detail? Formal operational? Dialectic/systemic?

_____

_____

_____

_____

almost complete. You receive additional and valuable information with which to more effectively work with your client. This information will assist you to more accurately determine your axis V Global Assessment of Functioning (GAF) score.

GOALS AND TREATMENT PLANS

Every helping professional must be able to design an effective treatment plan with appropriate goals. There are several components for developing accurate treatment plans, but the one cardinal rule seems quite simple: Devise your treatment plan and measurable goals around any or all of the above three strategies—stages of the interview, DSM-IV-TR axis, or developmental assessments. If you follow this formula, your counseling goals will assist you in implementation of that plan.

In designing your treatment plan and goals, first assess your problem list from the five DSM-IV-TR axes and/or the five stages of the interview as a way to organize a treatment plan. Look at your client's available resources and positive skills, and then identify the lack of meaningful activities, medical limitations, social isolation, and any suicidal ideations. Once your problem list is developed, you can begin to prioritize which needs must be addressed immediately, which needs could be addressed in the short term, and which issues will require long-term attention and goals (Ginter, 2002).

Remember, goals need to be set in behavioral terms that can be measurable. For example, with Susie, you could give her an assertiveness instrument to determine her basic communication skills. Administering the instrument could be a short-term goal. A long-term goal could be that in six months, the same instrument will be given to Susie. She will have increased her assertiveness rating by at least 10 points. Your goals are critical to the efficacy of the treatment. If you don't have goals, you cannot have direction for change.

CASE PRESENTATION GUIDELINES

Another important aspect of case conceptualization is the skills of presenting your client's case to other professionals. At the end of the chapter, Resource Q provides a sample outline that can assist you in putting all the information down concerning your client and the case study. Follow along using this outline as the Case of Rachel is used to demonstrate a narrative case presentation.

Narrative Case Presentation About Rachel

This is a concise example of a written case presentation about Rachel. Your instructor may want you to add more information, but you can use this format as a skeletal outline or guide. As you are reading this example narrative, think of other pertinent information that may need to go in this presentation. Remember that the purpose of a case presentation is to sufficiently advise others who may need to work with Rachel or to assist you in your treatment plan and supervisory needs.

I. Introduction

NAME AND PERSONAL INFORMATION: Rachel S. is a 71-year-old Caucasian woman whose presenting problem is sadness and anger about the death of her husband. She stated, "I just want my old life back." She displayed tangible signs of agitation, tearfulness, and depression. She appears to be stressed over issues of growing older and possibly losing her independence.

II. History

PRESENT PROBLEMS: Rachel stated the onset of her problems began when her husband, John, unexpectedly died six months ago of a heart attack.

Since that time Rachel reported, "I don't know what to do with myself." She does not eat or sleep regularly.

III. Past History of Psychiatric Illness: There is no reported past history of psychological illness.

IV. Contributing Medical Illness: From Rachel's Intake Form, the results of a recent physical showed high blood pressure. Rachel stated she was taking her blood pressure medicine on a daily basis.

V. Brief Family History: Her husband, John, died six months ago. They have three grown children who all live outside the state of Wyoming.

VI. Social History: Rachel and John were married 50 years. She is now a widow living on a fixed income, but John left her in a stable financial state. Rachel was a teacher and librarian for 30 years; both she and John had retired to travel and relax. She presently lives alone, but recently her children, especially the youngest child, are encouraging her to move away and live with one of them. Rachel believes she is very capable of living alone.

VII. DSM-IV Diagnosis

AXIS I: 309.0 Adjustment Disorder with Depressed Mood

AXIS II: 799.9 Deferred

AXIS III: 401.9 Hypertension/High Blood Pressure

AXIS IV: Bereavement; Children

AXIS V: GAF 70

VIII. Wellness Focus

(A) PHYSICAL: Rachel used to walk through the mall with her spouse three times a week. She is not exercising at all now. She maintains that her previous healthy eating habits are now sporadic. John loved to cook, and now Rachel hates cooking for one. Her sleep patterns are irregular.

(B) SPIRITUAL: According to Rachel's Intake Form, she belongs to a local First Methodist Church. She has been a member there for the past thirty years. She has not attended church since John's funeral.

(C) OCCUPATIONAL: Rachel is a retired teacher and librarian. Before John's death she was active in several local charity events, bridge, tutoring, and traveling.

(D) SOCIAL: Rachel reported that she and John had many friends and outlets for social activities. She has not contacted any friends since John's death.

(E) EMOTIONAL: Rachel labeled herself a happy person who enjoyed life. Her mother and father are both dead, and she remembers being sad but not devastated when they passed away. She remembered entering counseling one time when she lost her first baby, who was stillborn. Rachel said she only went a few times.

(F) INTELLECTUAL: Rachel stated she enjoys reading books and articles, both fiction and nonfiction. She discussed that lately she cannot focus long enough to read.

IX. Prognosis   Based on the Intake Form information and initial counseling interview, Rachel's counseling outcome and prognosis is good. If she continues to openly grieve the losses in her life and begins to create a new life without her husband, Rachel will develop the needed coping skills.

X. Treatment Goals in Specific and Measurable Terms   Four main counseling goals have been set with Rachel. Additional goals may be created as counseling continues.

1. Rachel will openly share her thoughts and feelings about her husband's death with her three children between now and the next two weeks.
2. Rachel will call at least one previous friend every week to arrange a social event.
3. Rachel will take a pre- and post-test Beck Depression Inventory to assess the degree of potential depression.
4. A Lifestyle Assessment Survey will be administered assessing wellness needs.

XI. Supervision Needs and Wants   During my individual and group supervision I would like for each of you in my supervisory group to watch for the following skills and problems:

1. Rachel seemed resistant in the very beginning of the counseling session. What could I have done differently to increase her level of comfort?
2. There were so many areas for us to focus on. I chose to focus on support resources. Was that the most effective and efficient area of focus?
3. The topic of death is not an easy issue for me. Did I handle my self-disclosure appropriately?
4. Please give me feedback on my five axes diagnosis.
5. What were my strengths? What could I improve upon?

Practical Reflection 4: Case Presentation Additions

As you read the case presentation, what would you add to the overall case study? What did you see as strengths in the presentation? What would you recommend for areas of development and improvement in the case presentation style?

_____

_____

_____

_____

THE CASE OF RACHEL: CASE CONCEPTUALIZATION WITH THE STAGES OF THE INTERVIEW, CLINICAL DIAGNOSIS, AND DEVELOPMENTAL ASSESSMENT

Stages of the Interview

Using the Stages of the Counseling Interview was helpful in comprehending the content and major concerns of Rachel. In the rapport/structuring stage, Rachel seemed resistant and stuck in her grief. Active listening skills were required. The exploration of concerns/data gathering stage revealed her additional concerns with her children and losing her independence. Stage three, mutual goal setting, assisted in developing the needed outcomes of counseling. The exploring alternatives stage assisted the case because available resources were discovered. Finally, the generalization and termination stage offered the necessary transitions for overcoming Rachel's grief and moving on to a new life.

DSM-IV-TR Diagnosis

A multiaxial diagnosis was offered in the narrative case presentation. An explanation of the diagnosis is offered, so you can dissect and compare the codes given for each axis.

DSM-IV-TR Axis I 309.00 Adjustment Disorder With Depressed Mood   Rachel came to counseling displaying symptoms of agitation,

sadness, loneliness, and confusion. During her interview, Rachel stated these symptoms had continued for a period of six months. For adjustment disorder to be considered, the client must exhibit marked distress in excess of what is expected and display significant social or occupational functioning. Bereavement was considered, as Rachel had valid and legitimate reasons for her grief, but her signs and symptoms seemed more intense than bereavement.

Axis II v799.9 Deferred Diagnosis   Rachel may have a personality disorder, but this axis diagnosis was deferred until tests can be given to substantiate or rule out any personality disorder.

Axis III 401.9 Hypertension   From the intake form and interview, Rachel disclosed that her high blood pressure or hypertension seems to be less manageable since her husband's death. Rachel must keep her blood pressure checked and under control to ensure that her medical condition does not interfere or contribute to the concerns in axis I.

Axis IV Bereavement and Concerns With Children   There were several psychosocial factors contributing to Rachel's primary counseling concern. In the counseling interview, Rachel discussed how lonely and sad she continues to be about John's death. She continues by disclosing that her children want her to move away and live with her youngest. These issues must be addressed during counseling as additional goals.

Axis V GAF 70   Assessing Rachel's overall functioning was relatively easy, as she was showing some signs and symptoms. In looking at the GAF continuum, the range of 61 to 70 stated, "Some mild symptoms or some difficulty in social, occupational, or school functioning, but generally functioning pretty well, has some meaningful interpersonal relationships"(APA, 1994, p.46). Rachel seemed to best fit into that range.

Developmental Assessment

Assessing Rachel's developmental needs seemed obvious as well. She spoke in analogies, such as "It is like my left arm has been cut off." Rachel preferred the D-3 orientation of patterns and analysis. Lori's comments matched Rachel's words; when summarizing, she commented, "a piece of you is missing." Lori continued to search for meaning, feelings, and themes for the remainder of the counseling session. Rachel was fairly independent, so Lori gave her intentional support, latitude, and a small amount of direct structure as they began goal setting.

Goals and Treatment for Rachel

The goals and treatment plan for Rachel may follow the multiaxial diagnosis and developmental assessment. As the treatment priority list is established, it is clear that Rachel is struggling with all the new transitions in her life. Learning about grief and openly sharing with her children was a priority in the short term.

Short-Term Goals

Goal 1. By the end of next week, Rachel will telephone each of her three children to talk about her grief and loneliness for their father.

Goal 2. By the end of next week, Rachel will tell her children about her feelings that they are coddling her.

Goal 3. By the end of next week, Rachel will call one friend to arrange a social outing.

Goal 4. By the end of the second counseling session, Rachel will have completed a Millon Clinical Multiaxial Inventory and a Beck Depression Inventory.

Long-Term Goals

Goal 1. By the end of one month, Rachel will have an appointment for a complete physical to check on her high blood pressure and to develop a baseline for physiologic needs.

Goal 2. By the fourth counseling session, Rachel and Lori will evaluate the previous goals for counseling outcomes and create new goals, if necessary.

Goal 3. By the eighth counseling session, Rachel will retake the Beck Depression Inventory for decrease in depression score.

Goal 4. As counseling progresses, Rachel will work on decision-making strategies for living arrangements, social activities, and projects.

These goals assist Lori in treating Rachel through this difficult period of adjustment to her husband's death. Because of Rachel's development levels, Lori will intentionally use encouragement and positive asset searches to guide Rachel. Gentle confrontations will challenge Rachel to stretch into an inclusive model of wellness.

SUMMARY AND PERSONAL INTEGRATION

The main emphasis of Chapter 5 was to create a better understanding of the steps involved in case conceptualization and treatment.

- We prescribed three strategies to assist in the case conceptualization process: stages of the interview, clinical diagnosis, and developmental assessment.
- Descriptions of the DSM-IV-TR axes were provided with examples of each.

Practical Reflection 5: Integration

As you read the material and reflections in Chapter 5, what aspects of case conceptualization will help you the most in effectively understanding your client's case and interventions?

_____

_____

_____

_____

- The Case of Rachel was presented to illustrate case conceptualization using the three strategies and emphasizing case presentation, goal setting, and treatment plans.

REFERENCES

American Psychiatric Association. (2000). *Diagnostic and Statistical Manual of Mental Disorders* (4th ed.), Text Revision. (DSM-IV-TR). Washington, DC: Author.

American Psychiatric Association. (1994). Desk Reference to the Diagnostic Criteria from DSM-IV. Text Modification. (DSM-IV-TM). Washington, DC: Author.

Ashen, A. (1977). *Psycheye: Self-Analytic Consciousness*. New York: Brandon House.

Bergman, J. S. (1985). *Fishing for Barracuda*. New York: WW Norton & Company.

Egan, G. (2002). The Skilled Helper (7th ed.). Pacific Grove, CA: Brooks/Cole.

Ginter, G. (2002). Treatment planning guidelines for children and adolescents. In R. R. Erk. (Ed.). *Counseling and Treatment for Children and Adolescents With DSM-IV-TR Disorders*. Upper Saddle River, NJ: Prentice Hall.

Hathaway, S. R., & McKinley, J. C. (1989). *Minnesota Multiphasic Personality Inventory-2*. Minneapolis: University of Minnesota; National Computer Systems.

Ivey, A., & Ivey, M. (1998). *Intentional Interviewing and Counseling* (4th ed.). Pacific Grove, CA: Brooks/Cole.

Ivey, A. E. & Ivey, M.B. (2003). *Intentional Interviewing and Counseling* (5th ed). Pacific Grove, CA: Brooks/Cole.

Kjos, D. (1994). What does DSM-IV have to do with counseling? *Illinois Counseling Association Quarterly, 133*, 2–10.

Millon, T. (1994). *Millon Clinical Multiaxial Inventory—III*. Minneapolis: National Computer Systems.

Smart, D., & Smart, J. (1997). DSM-IV and culturally sensitive diagnosis: Some observations for counselors. *Journal of Counseling and Development, 75*, 392–8.

United States Department of Health and Human Services. (2000). International Classification of Diseases. 10th Revision, Clinical Modification.

RESOURCE P

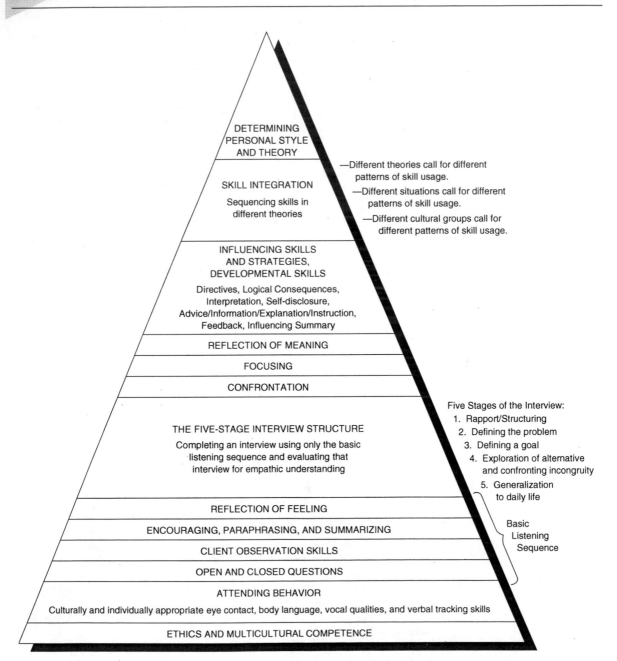

DETERMINING PERSONAL STYLE AND THEORY

SKILL INTEGRATION

Sequencing skills in different theories

—Different theories call for different patterns of skill usage.

—Different situations call for different patterns of skill usage.

—Different cultural groups call for different patterns of skill usage.

INFLUENCING SKILLS AND STRATEGIES, DEVELOPMENTAL SKILLS

Directives, Logical Consequences, Interpretation, Self-disclosure, Advice/Information/Explanation/Instruction, Feedback, Influencing Summary

REFLECTION OF MEANING

FOCUSING

CONFRONTATION

THE FIVE-STAGE INTERVIEW STRUCTURE

Completing an interview using only the basic listening sequence and evaluating that interview for empathic understanding

Five Stages of the Interview:
1. Rapport/Structuring
2. Defining the problem
3. Defining a goal
4. Exploration of alternative and confronting incongruity
5. Generalization to daily life

REFLECTION OF FEELING

ENCOURAGING, PARAPHRASING, AND SUMMARIZING

CLIENT OBSERVATION SKILLS

OPEN AND CLOSED QUESTIONS

Basic Listening Sequence

ATTENDING BEHAVIOR

Culturally and individually appropriate eye contact, body language, vocal qualities, and verbal tracking skills

ETHICS AND MULTICULTURAL COMPETENCE

RESOURCE Q

Case Presentation Outline Guide

   I. Introduction
       (a) Abbreviated Name of Client
       (b) Age
       (c) Gender
       (d) Presenting Problem(s) in Client's Words
       (e) Present Signs and Symptoms
       (f) Multicultural Domain Issues
  II. History
       (a) Present Problem(s)
           (1) Onset
           (2) Duration
 III. Past History of Psychiatric Illness
  IV. Contributing Medical Illness
   V. Brief Family History
  VI. Social History
       (a) Martial Status
       (b) Employment
       (c) Current Living Arrangements
 VII. DSM IV Diagnosis on five axes
       (a) Axis I: Presenting Problems and Focus of Clinical Attention
       (b) Axis II: Personality Disorders
       (c) Axis III: Relevant Medical Conditions
       (d) Axis IV: Psychosocial Stressors
       (e) Axis V: Global Affective Functioning (GAF)
VIII. Wellness Focus
       (a) Physical
       (b) Spiritual
       (c) Occupational
       (d) Social
       (e) Emotional
       (f) Intellectual
  IX. Prognosis
       (a) Poor
       (b) Fair
       (c) Good
   X. Treatment Goals in Specific and Measurable Terms
  XI. Student Counselor's Supervision Needs and Wants

KNOWLEDGE NEEDED TO GROW: ISSUES IN PROFESSIONAL PRACTICE

Chapter 6 is the beginning of Section Two and presents a third case study for you to analyze. The entire module addresses the myriad of issues facing a new helping professional. By the time you have completed Section Two and the remaining five chapters, you may expect to demonstrate:

- KNOWLEDGE AND COUNSELING SKILLS INVOLVED IN PRACTICING CULTURAL COMPETENCY.
- ATTITUDES AND BEHAVIORS NECESSARY FOR PROFESSIONAL AND ETHICAL COUNSELING.
- AN UNDERSTANDING OF OUTCOME RESEARCH AND ITS CORRELATION TO EFFECTIVE COUNSELING.
- A PHILOSOPHY OF WELLNESS, CREATING A PERSONAL AND PROFESSIONAL BALANCE.
- ADVOCACY FOR YOURSELF AND THE HELPING PROFESSION.

BECOMING A CULTURALLY COMPETENT HELPING PROFESSIONAL: APPRECIATION OF DIVERSITY

Knowing yourself well and becoming a culturally competent helping professional is a never-ending journey. It is a proactive and mindful process.

OVERVIEW

GOALS

KEY CONCEPTS: A CONTINUUM FOR MULTICULTURAL DEVELOPMENT

CROSS-CULTURAL DIMENSIONS IN COUNSELING
FAMILY CONTEXT
SOCIAL SYSTEMS CONTEXT
DEMOGRAPHIC CONTEXT
STATUS CONTEXT
LIFE EXPERIENCE CONTEXT
PRACTICAL REFLECTION 1: EXAMINING YOUR CULTURAL BELIEFS ABOUT HELPING

YOU AND MULTICULTURAL COMPETENCE
ATTITUDES AND BELIEFS GUIDELINES
PRACTICAL REFLECTION 2: INFLUENTIAL EXPERIENCES INFLUENCING YOUR CULTURAL IDENTITY
KNOWLEDGE GUIDELINES
PRACTICAL REFLECTION 3: STEREOTYPE DEVELOPMENT
SKILL GUIDELINES

PRACTICAL REFLECTION 4: PROACTIVE EXPERIENCES IN MULTICULTURAL DEVELOPMENT
MODELS OF RACIAL IDENTITY DEVELOPMENT
PRACTICAL REFLECTION 5: RACIAL IDENTITY DEVELOPMENT
AN EXAMPLE APPROACH FOR ENHANCING DIVERSITY APPRECIATION: A DIVERSITY SIMULATION
PRACTICAL REFLECTION 6: ALBATROSSIAN SIMULATION

EXAMPLE INTERVIEW: THE CASE OF DARRYL
THE CASE OF DARRYL
THE CASE OF DARRYL: A MULTICULTURAL PERSPECTIVE
PRACTICAL REFLECTION 7: RESPONSE TO THE CASE OF DARRYL

SUMMARY AND PERSONAL INTEGRATION
PRACTICAL REFLECTION 8: INTEGRATION

REFERENCES
RESOURCES R THROUGH T

OVERVIEW

Chapter 6 focuses on the need for multicultural competencies and encourages you to move from tolerance of differences to an appreciation of differences. Helping professionals must understand that diversity is inclusive of race, age, gender, sexual orientation, socioeconomic status, religious affiliation, and life experiences, and how each of these and other factors may impact the counseling process.

This chapter has several main emphases. The first goal is to provide you with a better understanding of your own beliefs and attitudes about living in a diverse society. Being aware of your personal worldview will affect how you engage in counseling. It is also imperative that you understand how stereotypes and prejudices occur. Several conceptual frameworks will be presented to assist you in comprehending the cross-cultural dynamics involved in counseling relationships (Kwan, 2001). Finally, you need to be aware of the many resources available to you in your diversity journey whether that be a diversity simulation or interacting with those who are different than you as in the Case of Darryl.

GOALS

1. Be aware of the Multicultural Competencies written for the helping professions.
2. Identify individual racial identities and prejudices.
3. Learn several Racial Identity Models.
4. Understand how multicultural dimensions affect diversity concerns.
5. React to a Diversity Simulation.
6. Analyze the Case of Darryl.

KEY CONCEPTS: A CONTINUUM FOR MULTICULTURAL DEVELOPMENT

It is crucial for you as a helping professional to have the awareness, knowledge, and skills to understand your own racial and cultural beliefs, values, and biases (Sue, Arredondo, & McDavis, 1992). If you understand yourself well, then you may be able to better assist in your client's development (Kwan, 2001). Helms (1995) noted that positive client change is more likely to occur if you are at a more advanced stage of racial identity development status than your client.

Once you understand your own racial development, you can apply the same three-stage model to your clients. According to Sue and Sue (1999), the first stage is Awareness. You must be aware that there are individual differences and be clear what your beliefs and values are. The second stage is Knowledge. You must gain needed information and knowledge about your client to help your client grow successfully. You must be able to "enter into the world of those you are trying to help by learning their unique cultures, family histories, languages, customs, values, and priorities" (Kottler, 2000, pp. 6–7). The third stage is Skills. There may be specific skills that work more sensitively and effectively with different types of concerns.

CROSS-CULTURAL DIMENSIONS IN COUNSELING

Cultural issues have become so broad that many believe all counseling is multicultural or cross cultural. Ivey, Pedersen, and Ivey (2001, pp. 2–3) classify the following factors to assist you in identifying essential multicultural dimensions.

Family Context

- Nuclear
- Extended family
- Adoptive
- Gay/lesbian
- Divorced
- Alcoholism/drugs

Social Systems Context

- Language
- Gender
- Ethnicity/race
- Religion and spirituality

Demographic Context

- Age
- Sexual orientation
- National origin
- Region of the nation
- Community of origin and present community

Practical Reflection 1: Examining Your Cultural Beliefs About Helping

What is your culture's existing way of helping? Answering that question is a start in understanding your own beliefs about helping. Discuss among your classmates.

_____

_____

_____

_____

Status Context

- Past and present socioeconomic background
- Education
- Key group affiliations (living group, fraternities, service agencies, athletics)

Life Experience Context

- Major physical issues
- Major emotional issues
- Experiences of discrimination or prejudice
- Experiences of trauma (rape, divorce, accident, serious illness, war)

Nwachuku and Ivey (1991) also believe that asking individuals from specific cultures to examine their own culture and describe the culture's values and helping styles is a beginning strategy for developing training materials for all helping professionals. As a student in field experience you can generalize this to working with individual clients, as well as better understanding your own personal helping style.

YOU AND MULTICULTURAL COMPETENCE

For years helping professionals have discussed the importance of using special skills when working with clients who are culturally different than the helper. It wasn't until the early 1990s that concerned multicultural leaders developed the Multicultural Competency Standards (Arredondo, Sue, & McDavis, 1992).

Multicultural counseling: Two or more persons who are working together in a counseling relationship presenting differing ways of perceiving the world and environment.

Multicultural Counseling Competencies and Standards: A set of standards for working with clients of minority populations.

The competencies presented below have been endorsed by many professional helping groups, among them the Association for Multicultural Counseling and Development, the Association for Counselor Education and Supervision, and the Counseling Psychology division of the American Psychological Association. At this writing the competencies are being reviewed by the American Psychological Association as guidelines for professional practice, research and teaching. Social work and human services have their own approaches to these key issues.

Using the Multicultural Competency Standards developed by Sue, Arredondo, and McDavis (1992); Kwan (2001) developed the following guidelines to assist you in exploring your personal multicultural journey. Read through each sentence and first decide whether you agree or disagree with the guideline and what it means to you. If you believe the guideline is true or useful for you, then begin to dissect how it might play a role in your work with clients.

Attitudes and Beliefs Guidelines

Culturally Skilled Counselors Believe That Cultural Self-Awareness and Sensitivity to One's Own Cultural Heritage Is Essential. Every Person Has a Culture.   Examine your own culture and begin to recognize what influences that may have on your development. For example, our children go to a school where diversity is valued. My nine-year-old is having a birthday party next week. I told him he could invite four other children. His best buddy is African American and his second best buddy is Vietnamese. Jaimeson's worldview is very different than mine as a child.

Culturally Skilled Counselors Are Aware of How Their Own Cultural Background and Experiences Have Influenced Attitudes, Values, and Biases About Psychological Processes.   Look at yourself as a multicultural being—race/ethnicity, spirituality, gender, sexual orientation, and so on. All these variables play a role in how you see the world. Defining the world in this manner, it is easy to depict all counseling as multicultural.

One of my most pivotal experiences as a teenager was to travel to New York City and be a part of the annual United Nations Pilgrimage! It was then that I realized that the world is vast and made up of many different populations and traditions. As I interacted with others who were different than I, the realization hit me that still we are more alike than different!

Culturally Skilled Counselors Are Able to Recognize the Limits of Their Multicultural Competency and Expertise.   As you think about

---

Practical Reflection 2: Influential Experiences Influencing Your Cultural Identity

You need to familiarize and assess your own personal ideas about all of the attitudes and beliefs, knowledge, and skills guidelines. For now, please select at least one personal response that you would be willing to share with your classmates. For example, what cultural background and experiences have influenced you and your beliefs about people and the psychological processes?

_____

_____

_____

_____

---

the varying cultural groups reviewed, how much knowledge and experience have you had with each group? Recognizing your limitations in certain areas is important. Asking others to help you learn more is a compliment to that group. Most people love to share information about their beliefs and cultural traditions.

Knowledge Guidelines

Culturally Skilled Counselors Have Specific Knowledge About Their Own Racial and Cultural Heritage and How It Personally and Professionally Affects Their Definitions of and Biases About Normality/Abnormality and the Process of Counseling. If you haven't already done so, this is a great opportunity to learn more about your cultural heritage. Dissect your cultural dimensions and see how they have affected you, positively and negatively. How has your ethnic background influenced you? What has your religious/spiritual background given you? Are your beliefs yours alone, or do you share them with your parents and grandparents?

A favorite anecdote demonstrates how traditions and beliefs are passed down through the ages. It goes something like this. A newly wed couple is preparing their first Sunday afternoon dinner. It is a pot roast with tasty vegetables. The husband carefully observes his wife's detailed preparation. Just before placing the roast in the pan, she takes a large knife and cuts off the end of the meat. In conversation, the husband asks

Practical Reflection 3: Stereotype Development

Based on the knowledge from this chapter and your own personal experiences, how have many of your stereotypes developed? Every one has biases and prejudices. Try discussing yours with your classmates and/or supervisor.

_____

_____

_____

_____

his wife why she cut off the end of the meat. She replies, "I don't truly know, but my mother always does that!" The curious wife calls her mother and inquires. Her mother says, "I don't truly know, but my mother always does that!" Luckily for our story, the grandmother is still living! Grandmother is asked why she cuts off the end of the meat. The grandmother begins to laugh, "Honey, I cut off the end of the meat because my pan was way too little for the roast!"

Culturally Skilled Counselors Possess Knowledge and Understanding About How Oppression, Racism, Discrimination, and Stereotyping Affect Them Personally and in Their Work.   It is important for you to discuss and understand your own situations with oppression, stereotyping, and so on. All of us have experienced some aspect of discrimination. The frequency of the events and your responses and reactions to them help you to better understand the process of oppression. Understanding is the first step; acting and choosing to intervene on the process is another phase.

Culturally Skilled Counselors Possess Knowledge About Their Social Impact on Others. They Are Knowledgeable About Communication Style Differences, How Their Style May Clash With or Foster the Counseling Process With Persons of Color or Those Different From Themselves and How to Anticipate the Impact It May Have on Others.   In several of the previous chapters, you have been encouraged to ask for feedback during your supervision sessions. Your supervision is a wonderful opportunity to ask others you trust about your social impact on

---

Practical Reflection 4: Proactive Experiences in Multicultural Development

What have you done in the past and what are you doing presently to become skilled as a multicultural helping professional?

_____

_____

_____

_____

---

others. Supervision provides a relatively safe environment to discuss your reactions and responses to those who are different. Each of us do tend to react in our own style to differences.

Skill Guidelines

Culturally Skilled Counselors Seek Out Educational, Consultative, and Training Experiences to Improve Their Understanding and Effectiveness in Working With Culturally Different Populations. If you believe this guideline is true, then demonstrate your belief through your actions by doing something to improve your understanding and effectiveness. If you have not taken a course on diversity, this is the time. Attending a diversity fair, going out to lunch with someone who is different from you, and having a party with a diverse group of people are steps in the right direction.

Culturally Skilled Counselors Are Constantly Seeking to Understand Themselves as Racial and Cultural Beings and Are Actively Seeking a Nonracist and Nonoppressive Identity. You have a chance to demonstrate your opposition to discrimination of any type. Be sure to work with others to fight against it. You can begin small by not laughing at an insensitive joke or asserting your thoughts during a meeting where an oppressive statement was made. Again begin with small gestures to spread the word against discrimination.

Models of Racial Identity Development

Three models will be presented to assist you in better understanding the manner in which racial identities may be developed. As you read each model, integrate the previous information into this material on racial identity development.

People of Color Racial Identity Developmental Model   Helms described five ego identity statuses in the People of Color Racial Identity Developmental Model (POC/RID): (1) Conformity, where you believe that other cultures are superior; (2) Encounter/dissonance, when a racial situation causes dissonance of previously held beliefs; (3) Immersion/ emersion, when identified culture is idealized and White culture is criticized; (4) Internalization, when reappraisals of selective cultures are organized; and (5) Integration, when you becomes less reactive and the identity comprises the benefits of cultures involved. Integration allows you to make a commitment to advocate against any kind of racial discrimination.

White Racial Identity Developmental Model   In the White Racial Identity Developmental Model (W/RID) you would go through a series of ego statuses or expressions of current racial identity. Each status has an Information Processing Strategy (IPS) that allows you to reflect on the information given that is race related. The information could be attitudinal, behavioral, or affective. If you are White, Helms stated that moving through the six statuses requires an awareness first that racism does exists and then "abandonment of entitlement" and personal superiority must be addressed (Helms, 1995, p. 184).

During Abandonment of Racism, there are three statuses involved on the continuum: (1) Contact with others and recognition of racism; (2) Disintegration of current beliefs about diversity and guilt surrounding racial issues; and (3) Reintegration, which includes idealization of White status and confusion with racial issues.

In the second phase, you become more actively involved in Defining a Nonracist Identity. There are three statuses in which you must evolve: (1) Pseudoindependence from your race but still a cognitive commitment to your race; (2) Immersion/emersion, which may include racial activism; and (3) Autonomy, which allows you to move away from your privileged status and work toward the benefits of a diverse society.

Helms Racial Identity Interaction Process Model   Helms (1995) emphasizes even more the importance of your knowing your own racial identity status, because it does interact with the racial identity status of your client. Helms and Cook (1999) believe that the "counselor's expression of her or his underlying racial identity statuses influences his or her reaction to the client, and the client's underlying statuses, in turn, influences his or her reactions to the counselor" (p. 180). Pederson (2002) articulates that you have thousands of "culture teachers" such as friends, family, enemies,

---

Practical Reflection 5: Racial Identity Development

After reading the three racial identity models, select one model that fits you and discuss your own racial development.

_____

_____

_____

_____

---

and images that continually influence your racial identity. It is a mistake not to recognize these internalized influences.

Helms (1995) postulates that there are three possible, distinct counseling relationships that can occur as racial identity statuses emerge: (1) parallel, (2) regressive, and (3) progressive. Parallel relationships occur when the helping professional and client have similar worldviews. The opposite happens in regressive counseling relationships, where the client has a more mature racial identity than the counselor and conflicts continue to erupt. The final progressive relationship occurs when the helping professional has a more advanced racial identity than the client. Although this counseling relationship can still have challenges and conflict, the counselor can more readily facilitate growth in the client.

An Example Approach for Enhancing Diversity Appreciation: A Diversity Simulation

According to Russell and Berger (1993), diversity simulations can be powerful and effective tools for teaching people to discover personal attitudes toward inclusivity. Often when you engage in multicultural trainings, much needed information is given, but there seems to be few "activating events" to get you out of the intellectual viewing of diversity and into your own personal worldview (Russell-Chapin & Stoner, 1995).

One of the main reasons simulations work is that you are given no verbal instructions or information about the experience, so you must use your own worldview to make meaning of the simulation. Frequently, the only way to make meaning is to enter the experience with preconceived perceptions from prior life experiences and filters.

There is a simulation that we use in the classroom and during consultations, and every time people react in the same way. They are surprised, angry, curious, confused, and embarrassed! A classic diversity simulation is called "The Albatross" created by Batchelder and Warner (1977). Russell-Chapin and Stoner (1995) emphasize the need for ambiguity when presenting the Albatrossian simulation. The less information that is provided, the more you have to rely on your own filters to understand this ambiguous situation.

Imagine this experience for yourself.

You walk into a dimly lit room where a woman dressed in an ornate gown is sitting on the floor. A man is sitting in a chair next to her. There are four more empty chairs arranged in a semi-circle. A candle and incense are burning and unique music is playing quietly. The entire environmental setup is different and out of character and context.

The man rises and begins to select male participants. There are no verbal instructions or words spoken. The men are individually directed to sit in chairs. The head male grunts to each man to sit. He then sits and makes four clicking noises. The woman rises to her feet and she begins to select women to join the group. Each woman is nonverbally asked to come, but before sitting on the floor, shoes must be removed and placed beneath the chairs.

The head male grunts again and demonstrates how to place their hands on the women's head and push the heads to the floor. The participants imitate the facilitator and push the head to the floor of the female kneeling to their right.

Another set of clicking noises is heard and the head woman rises and brings a bowl of water. Each man must wash their hands, but the women do not.

There is a head pushing at the end of each aspect of the tradition.

Next the head facilitator clicks and the head woman quickly responds by feeding each male an unfamiliar edible food with a toothpick. It is served by the head female. Then the women all eat but they serve themselves.

A similar round of events happens with drinking from one chalice. The head female serves the cup to the lips of the males, while the females all drink the unique liquid one by one.

The final component of the simulation occurs when the male clicks and both rise. The women are directed to display their feet and the two facilitators walk around observing the women's feet. One woman is selected and directed to rise. She is joined with the head male and they walk outside!

Following the simulation, the processing of the experiences begins. The facilitators offer a four-tiered system of organizing the activating event. First you are asked to describe what each of you actually observed.

Practical Reflection 6: Albatrossian Simulation

As you read the Albatrossian script, what were your first impressions? How were you feeling?

_____

_____

_____

_____

Inevitably people respond by interpreting what the performance meant, not describing what they saw or observed. For example, you might say the performance was an example of subservience of women rather than describing that men sat on chairs and the women sat on the floor.

Once the group understands how to describe actual events and not first react with emotions and assumptions, then the facilitators move to the second tier.

In this next part of the discussion, you are asked to share how the performance made you feel. Typically, many people from the group, whether they are participants or observers, are uncomfortable, angry, and confused. The third tier asks for a discussion of meaning. Usually the group states that it is a ritual of some sort where men are dominant and women are inferior.

Finally, the facilitators reveal that this simulation represents a demonstration of a matriarchal society, not a patriarchal one. Uniformly, there is surprise, confusion, and embarrassment! According to Russell-Chapin and Stoner (1995),

> Most individuals desire immediate answers (to unfamiliar events) and ascribing interpretation or meaning from individual perceptual sets provides more comfort and security. What they do not acknowledge or realize is that this interpretation is filtered from personal perceptual sets and frequently is not accurate for another culture or person. When participants take the risk to describe accurately what was seen, they are ready to take the next step by asking questions about possible meanings. (p. 152)

The facilitators assist each of you to then go through the first three tiers of the organization system to describe what you saw and make that perceptual switch, now that you know it is an example of a matriarchal system. Each observation can be taken one by one and processed. For example, why would men be fed with toothpicks and not the women? Possibly, the men must be fed first to ensure that the food is safe, so that the women can eat it! The perceptual switch can be made for each observation.

The Albatrossian Simulation is just one category of activating events, but any activity that can assist you or others to "get out of your heads and into your personal belief system" is a powerful mechanism to learn and integrate diversity into your life. These types of experiences can become catalyst for change and are a must if diversity is to be lived and acted upon (Russell-Chapin & Stoner, 1995). In the next section, your second case study will unfold. Take risks as you read the case study. Begin to see how understanding diversity will assist you in better serving this client.

EXAMPLE INTERVIEW: THE CASE OF DARRYL

Darryl was introduced to you in the Preface. You may want to review his history again. He entered Lori's life much later in her professional counseling career. Their first counseling encounter had Darryl in a dissociative state with only a small amount of the initial counseling interview occurring. Lori did join Darryl on the floor, and toward the end of the session they processed the happenings of the first meeting. Darryl requested a second appointment two days later. Darryl is a 45-year-old African American man.

We are presenting your third case study in this chapter for two reasons. Begin viewing the Case of Darryl with a cumulative perspective from chapters 1 through 5, plus add to your worldview the ideas of additional related multicultural issues.

You may want to use another CIRF and continue to classify and process the interviewing skills. There is a blank copy of the CIRF in Resource R. Again, you are welcome to compare your classifications with our CIRF in Resource S. See Resource T for the entire script with skill identifications. Be sure to begin to view the Cases of Stephen and Rachel from a multicultural aspect as well.

The Case of Darryl

(1) LORI: *Hi, Darryl, I am glad you came today.*
(2) DARRYL: *Me, too, I guess.*
(3) LORI: *From your voice and posture, you sound a bit ambivalent about being here.*
(4) DARRYL: *I do want to be here because I have so much to share, but I can't believe I was so scared that I began talking in*

tongues. I do that sometimes. My father was an evangelist. I am glad I didn't scare you off.

(5) LORI: You didn't scare me off. I know very little about talking in tongues. You may have to teach me more, but the two of us can make this a safe place to discuss anything you want. Last time I didn't take the time to explain how I do counseling. Perhaps this would be a good time.

(6) DARRYL: Yes, I want to know more about the way you do counseling. So far, you are doing OK. You know, I have seen lots of other professionals, so I probably know the scoop. I like the fact you were sitting on the floor with me last time, though.

(7) LORI: I appreciate your giving me feedback, Darryl. As I will do the same with you. The more the two of us can become a team and build a counseling relationship, the better your counseling will go.

(8) DARRYL: You want me to work with you? Maybe I don't know the scoop, cuz most of the time people just tell me what to do.

(9) LORI: Darryl, I will not tell you what to do. My job is to listen to your concerns and assist you with your desired changes. I do not have the answers, but I can help you through the process of change.

(10) DARRYL: I thought you would have the answers!

(11) LORI: You have the answers, Darryl, to your problems. I can help you discover the needed answers by guiding you to the many possible solutions.

(12) DARRYL: I would like to find some solutions. I seem to have lots of problems.

(13) LORI: We all have problems, Darryl. Let's talk about your problems today, and by the end of this session, we will set several counseling goals to give us some counseling direction. How does that sound to you?

(14) DARRYL: Strange, but good.

(15) LORI: Darryl, what do you want to work on today in counseling?

(16) DARRYL: My life seems to be falling apart. I am struggling in my marriage, and I am having a difficult time keeping my job intact. The most frustrating thing is that I have been in this place before.

(17) LORI: You are explaining to me that your marital problems and job difficulties are not new experiences. How discouraging that must be.

(18) DARRYL: Yes, it is. It is deeper than discouragement, though, this time it seems hopeless.

(19) LORI: I am sorry, Darryl, that you are in such a desperate place in your life. (Reflection of Meaning)

(20) DARRYL: Thanks for being so kind and understanding. My wife, Sophia, thinks I am a bum. This is the third job I have had since our marriage of seven years. Our son, Michael, is four, and he loves to draw pictures. He drew a picture of me. I don't know exactly what it means, but his depiction of me made me very sad. He drew me shouting with a mouthful of teeth.

(21) LORI: What ever is happening in your life is keeping you from having a healthy marriage and job. Sophia finds your work history unreliable, and Michael thinks you are angry some of the time. Is that correct?

(22) DARRYL: Absolutely correct.

(23) LORI: What do you want to do about all this, Darryl?

(24) DARRYL: I don't know. You are the counselor, you tell me.

(25) LORI: It probably would be easier, if I could tell you what to do, but I can't, Darryl. Remember I don't have the answers to your life.

(26) DARRYL: Now you are not being helpful.

(27) LORI: Help comes in many forms. If all your old ways of thinking and feelings have not worked, then let's try a different approach. Darryl, tell me the last time your life was not falling apart.

(28) DARRYL: (There is a long pause, and Darryl begins to stare. I thought he might go into another trance-like, dissociative state.)

(29) LORI: Darryl, it is okay if you need to go away. I will be here when you get back. You need to know that you are safe in here.

(30) DARRYL: (After several minutes of silence) I have been going away for many years. Sophia hates it and screams at me.

(31) LORI: My guess is that Sophia may be scared too and doesn't know what to do either.

(32) DARRYL: I think she just hates me because I am a no-good bum.

(33) LORI: Darryl, I appreciate your choosing, on some level, not to dissociate. That makes our work here easier. You will be okay in here. Let's focus again on a time when your life was not falling apart.

(34) DARRYL: Well, it was many years ago. I had decided that I would be single forever. I had my dog, Alex, and a good job as a nurse practitioner. My past was behind me. I felt good helping others and working in a doctor's office.

(35) LORI: I want to make sure I understand. Years ago, you re-membered a time when your life was together. You enjoyed your

single lifestyle, your dog, Alex, and your nursing job. Helping other people seemed the right thing to do. Is that accurate?

(36) DARRYL: *Yes. Even hearing you talk about my old life makes me happy and sad.*

(37) LORI: *There are those ambivalent feelings again, Darryl. Life has both happy and sad, doesn't it?*

(38) DARRYL: *Yes, but I hate sad times.*

(39) LORI: *What do you hate about sad times, Darryl?*

(40) DARRYL: *In my life there have been more sad times than not.*

(41) LORI: *(I decided to be silent for at least two minutes!) What were some of your saddest times, Darryl?*

(42) DARRYL: *(Tears were welling in his eyes.) My sad times are too sad to share!*

(43) LORI: *You do not have to share them, Darryl. (We sat in silence).*

(44) DARRYL: *I want to share them with you, though.*

(45) LORI: *You are being very brave, Darryl. Tell me about your sad times.*

(46) DARRYL: *I was a medic in Viet Nam. I saw such devastation, but I honestly was doing okay. Knowing I was being helpful seemed to make the atrocities a little better. I helped many people, and I saw many men die.*

(47) LORI: *I can't imagine what you saw and lived through, but the fact that you saved so many people helped you through many difficult times.*

(48) DARRYL: *I guess so. One night my best friend, Stan, and I were together. Stan didn't have many friends and he was kind of little. The other guys made fun of him. I really liked Stan. His friendship made the war more tolerable.*

(49) LORI: *Sounds as if you were a very good friend and that you helped people in many different ways.*

(50) DARRYL: *NO! I was not a good friend. I am done here. I need to go!*

(51) LORI: *Darryl, if you need to go, you can. Before you go, I want to give you an observation. When you were talking of Stan initially, your voice was soft and almost dreamy. When I suggested that you were a good friend to Stan, your voice became loud and aggressive. What are those voice changes about?*

(52) DARRYL: *I really need to go away.*

(53) LORI: *It is okay that you go. We will see each other again. There are many ways of "going away," aren't there, Darryl?*

(54) DARRYL: *You are really a pain in the neck.*

(55) LORI: *I can be a pain in the neck. I believe I am in good hands, though.*

(56) DARRYL: Okay, I won't go away, but you are not in good hands.

(57) LORI: You sound like a very competent nurse and friend, Darryl. Tell me why I am not in good hands.

(58) DARRYL: (Darryl begins shouting.) You are not in good hands, because these hands did not stop things I should have stopped. Are you happy now!

(59) LORI: I am not happy, Darryl, but I truly appreciate continuing to talk to me about such difficult times.

(60) DARRYL: I don't like to talk about my past. I haven't spoke a word of it to anyone, not even to my wife, Sophia.

(61) LORI: Then many memories are buried very deep.

(62) DARRYL: (Darryl begins to weep.)

(63) LORI: This must be very painful and devastating.

(64) DARRYL: It is more than devastating. It should not have happened. For years I wished I had been able to stop the hurt that we caused so many people.

(65) LORI: So for all these past years, you have carried around the burdens that you saw.

(66) DARRYL: Yes, I feel guilty for living. I have moments when I am happy with Sophia and Michael, but they are fleeting.

(67) LORI: Tell me what you should have stopped.

(68) DARRYL: One night, Stan and I were in a village and we heard sobbing and screaming. We approached the huts carefully and saw our own soldiers raping the village women. Stan and I told them to stop, but several of the men yelled at us to get lost and mind our own business. That night I went back to our temporary quarters, and I began having horrible nightmares! Those dreams still haunt me.

(69) LORI: That must have been frightening. And I would like to hear about your dreams, Darryl.

(70) DARRYL: That is just it. I am not sure they were dreams.

(71) LORI: What do you mean you are not sure they were dreams?

(72) DARRYL: This is so difficult to say...I have been trying to piece together things.

(73) LORI: Tell me about those things, Darryl.

(74) DARRYL: Well, I believe someone close to me sexually hurt me as a child. Bits and pieces come back to me, whether it be in dreams or vivid pictures in my head. I just don't know.

(75) LORI: There are so many of the dreams and pictures in your head that you believe they might be connected to a time when someone may have sexually hurt you. Is that right?

(76) DARRYL: *I think so.*

(77) LORI: *Is it possible that the night in Viet Nam triggered some of your current behaviors and feelings?*

(78) DARRYL: *I hadn't put the two together, but it makes some sense, as that is when the dreams began. I just don't want to believe that someone close could sexually harm me.*

(79) LORI: *You and I do not know if that is true or not. We may never know the truth, but that is not the issue here. Whether sexual abuse occurred or not is not the problem. We need to create a way for you to handle your present situation and your many perceptions about your past. Since we cannot change the past, one of our counseling goals is to change your perceptions of that past. That we can do.*

(80) DARRYL: *That doesn't sound easy.*

(81) LORI: *It is not easy, but we can do it together as a team. How does that sound to you?*

(82) DARRYL: *Nothing else has been working, so it is worth a try. Where do we start?*

(83) LORI: *You and I have already started, Darryl. You will never be the same again, you have bravely faced the beast today in whatever form it appears.*

(84) DARRYL: *It feels like such a long haul.*

(85) LORI: *It will be worth your effort, Darryl. The outcome may be that you learn new coping mechanisms to deal with your past and present.*

(86) DARRYL: *I want my life to be different. I want Sophia and Michael to have a husband and father who can cope better with what ever life brings.*

(87) LORI: *I believe you can do that, Darryl. You even coped differently here. Talk to me about how you coped differently today.*

(88) DARRYL: *(a long silence) I guess I did cope differently today. I felt strong enough to tell you things I have never shared . . . and I somehow did not "go away" when you asked me difficult questions.*

(89) LORI: *So you have at least two new coping skills to take with you to assist in the week to come. As a homework assignment for the next week, please share with Sophia whatever comes into your mind. I have a feeling she will appreciate sharing more than "going away." Also please spend at least 15 minutes a day with Michael doing some fun activity.*

(90) DARRYL: *What if I shout at Michael again?*

(91) LORI: *You will shout again, but this time Michael will also have quality time to remember. Darryl, how committed are you to these two homework goals?*

(92) DARRYL: *I believe I can accomplish these two goals by sharing with Sophia and playing more with Michael.*
(93) LORI: *So you are committed to these goals. Before we go, I want to ask one more question. What kind of nurse were you in counseling today?*
(94) DARRYL: *That is a funny question . . . but I guess I was a helpful and brave medic and nurse.*
(95) LORI: *You applied your skills as a helping nurse practitioner to yourself! Wow! You shared and faced your fears. Darryl, when do you want to come back to counseling?*
(96) DARRYL: *Do you have something available early in the week?*
(97) LORI: *There's an opening on Tuesday. See you at 10:00. Enjoy those competent nursing skills.*

Darryl and Lori continued to counsel together over a period of two years. During that time Darryl was hospitalized once for severe depression. Working conjointly with a psychiatrist, Darryl was placed on an antidepressant, and then continued in counseling with Lori. His prognosis was good, and he went back to work as a nurse practitioner.

The Case of Darryl: A Multicultural Perspective

As you begin to analyze the Case of Darryl, many of the dimensions suggested in this chapter come to life. Darryl and Lori had to understand the differences of race, gender, age, life experiences, religion, and coping strategies.

It has been suggested that you need to address the racial differences soon after developing a counseling relationship (Sanders-Thompson, 1994). Notice that Lori did address the differences between religious

---

Practical Reflection 7: Response to the Case of Darryl

After reading the script from the Case of Darryl, describe your thoughts and feelings concerning the cultural differences between Darryl and Lori. Share your responses with your colleagues.

_____

_____

_____

_____

experiences in the beginning of the session. Review the script beginning with statement number 5.

Soon after Lori chose to begin working on the symptoms that were debilitating Darryl the most. Once Darryl's symptoms of depression and dissociation were addressed and maintained, Lori and Darryl began work on racial identity concerns together.

SUMMARY AND PERSONAL INTEGRATION

In this chapter you were introduced to several approaches for assisting you in becoming a culturally competent helping professional:

- Multicultural dimensions and multicultural competencies were presented to assist you in better understanding yourself and counseling others.
- Models of racial identity and the interaction process between client and helping professional were described.
- An example of an educational diversity simulation was presented.
- The third case study of the book was presented to continue demonstrating the variety of issues facing you on your helping professional journey.

Practical Reflection 8: Integration

What Chapter 6 constructs, models, and/or techniques will assist you the most in becoming a culturally competent helping professional?

_____

_____

_____

_____

REFERENCES

Batchelder, D., & Warner, E. (Eds.). (1997). *Beyond Experience: The Experiential Approach to Cross-Cultural Education.* Brattleboro, VT: Experiment Press.

Helms J. E. (1995). An update of Helm's white and people of color racial identity models. In J. G. Ponterotto, J. M. Casas, L. A. Suzuki, & C. M. Alexander (Eds.). *Handbook of Multicultural Counseling* (pp. 181–91). Thousand Oaks, CA: Sage.

Helms, J. E., & Cook, D. A. (1999). *Using Race and Culture in Counseling and Psychotherapy: Theory and Process*. Needham Heights, MA: Allyn & Bacon.

Ivey, A., Pedersen, P., & Ivey, M. (2001). *Intentional Group Counseling*. Pacific Grove, CA: Brooks/Cole.

Kottler, J. (2000). *Nuts and Bolts of Helping*. Boston, MA: Allyn & Bacon.

Kwan, K. K. (2001). Models of racial and ethnic identity development: Delineation of practical implications. *Journal of Mental Health Counseling, 23*, 269–77.

Nwachuku, U. T., & Ivey, A. E. (1991). Culture-specific counseling: An alternative training model. *Journal of Counseling and Development, 70*, 106–11.

Pederson, P. (2002). In F. D. Harper & J. McFadden (Eds.). *Culture and Counseling: New Approaches*. New York: New York: Pearson Education.

Russell, L. A., & Berger, S. (1993). Learning about diversity: A multicultural simulation. *Journal of College Student Development, 34*, 438–9.

Russell-Chapin, L. A., & Stoner, C. (1995). Mental health consultants for diversity training. *Journal of Mental Health Counseling, 17*, 146–55.

Sanders-Thompson, V. (1994). A preliminary outline of treatment strategies with African Americans coping with racism. *Psychological Discourse, 25*, 6–9.

Sue, D. W., Arredondo, P., & McDavis, R. J.(1992). Multicultural competencies/standards: A call to the profession. *Journal of Counseling and Development, 70*, 477–86.

Sue, D. W., & Sue, D. (1999). *Counseling the Culturally Different: Theory and Practice*. (3rd Ed.). New York: Wiley.

RESOURCE R

COUNSELING INTERVIEW RATING FORM

Counselor: _____   Date: _____
Observer: _____   Tape Number: _____
Observer: _____   Audio or video (please circle)
Supervisor: _____   Session Number:_____

For each of the following specific criteria demonstrated, make a frequency marking every time the skill is demonstrated. Then assign points for consistent skill mastery using the ratings scales below. Active mastery of each skill receives a score of 2. Skills marked with an X should be seen consistently on every tape. List any observations, comments, strengths and weaknesses in the space provided. Providing actual counselor phrases is helpful when offering feedback.

Ivey Mastery Ratings

3   Teach the skill to clients (teaching mastery only)
2   Use the skill with specific impact on client (active mastery)
1   Use and/or identify the counseling skill (basic mastery)
    To receive an A on a tape at least 52–58 points must be earned.
    To receive a B on a tape at least 46–51 points must be earned.
    To receive a C on a tape at least 41–45 points must be earned.

Specific Criteria		Frequency	Comments	Skill Mastery Rating
A. Opening/developing rapport				
1. Greeting	X			
2. Role definition/expectation				
3. Administrative tasks				
4. Beginning	X			
B. Exploration phase/ defining the problem micro skills				
1. Empathy/rapport				
2. Respect				
3. Nonverbal matching	X			
4. Minimal encourager	X			
5. Paraphrasing	X			
6. Pacing/leading	X			
7. Verbal tracking	X			
8. Reflect feeling	X			
9. Reflect meaning	X			
10. Clarifications	X			
11. Open-ended questions	X			

(continued)

RESOURCE R CONTINUED

Specific Criteria	Frequency	Comments	Skill Mastery Rating
12. Summarization	X		
13. Behavioral description	X		
14. Appropriate closed question	X		
15. Perception check	X		
16. Silence	X		
17. Focusing	X		
18. Feedback	X		
C. Problem-solving skills/ defining skills			
1. Definition of goals	X		
2. Exploration/understanding of concerns	X		
3. Development/evaluation of alternatives	X		
4. Implement alternative			
5. Special techniques			
6. Process counseling			
D. Action phase/ confronting incongruities			
1. Immediacy			
2. Self-disclosure			
3. Confrontation			
4. Directives			
5. Logical consequences			
6. Interpretation			
E. Closing/generalization			
1. Summarization of content/feeling	X		
2. Review of plan	X		
3. Rescheduling			
4. Termination of session			
5. Evaluation of session	X		
6. Follow-up			
F. Professionalism			
1. Developmental level match			
2. Ethics			
3. Professional (punctual, attire, etc.)			
G. Strengths:			
Area for Improvement:			

Total _____

RESOURCE S

COUNSELING INTERVIEW RATING FORM

Counselor: <u>Lori Russell-Chapin</u>   Date: <u>November, 2002</u>

Observer: _____   Tape Number: <u>2</u>

Observer: _____   Audio or Video; please circle

Supervisor: <u>Allen Ivey</u>   Session Number: <u>II</u>

For each of the following specific criteria demonstrated, make a frequency marking every time the skill is demonstrated. Then assign points for consistent skill mastery using the ratings scales below. Active mastery of each skill receives a score of 2. Skills marked with an X should be seen consistently on every tape. List any observations, comments, strengths and weaknesses in the space provided. Providing actual counselor phrases is helpful when offering feedback.

Ivey Mastery Ratings

3   Teach the skill to clients (teaching mastery only)
2   Use the skill with specific impact on client (active mastery)
1   Use and/or identify the counseling skill (basic mastery)
    To receive an A on a tape, at least 52–58 points must be earned.
    To receive a B on a tape, at least 46–51 points must be earned.
    To receive a C on a tape, at least 41–45 points must be earned.

Specific Criteria		Frequency	Comments	Skill Mastery Rating
A. Opening/developing rapport				
1. Greeting	X	I	"Hi, Darryl, I am glad you came today."	2
2. Role definition/ expectation		I	"I appreciate your giving me feedback, Darryl. As I will do the same with you. The more the two of us can become a team and build a counseling relationship, the better your counseling will go."	2
3. Administrative tasks				
4. Beginning	X	I	"Darryl, what do you want to work on today in counseling?"	2
B. Exploration phase/ defining the problem microskills		III	"Darryl, it is okay if you need to go away. I will be here when you get back. You need to know that you are safe in here."	2
1. Empathy/rapport				
2. Respect				
3. Nonverbal matching	X			
4. Minimal encourager	X			

(*continued*)

RESOURCE S CONTINUED

Specific Criteria		Frequency	Comments	Skill Mastery Rating
5. Paraphrasing	X	IIII	"So for all these past years, you have carried around the burdens that you saw."	2
6. Pacing/Leading	X	II	"We all have problems, Darryl. Let's talk about your problems today, and by the end of this session, we will set several counseling goals to give us some counseling direction. How does that sound to you?"	2
7. Verbal tracking	X	III	"You didn't scare me off. The two of us can make this a safe place to discuss anything you want. Last time I didn't take the time to explain how I do counseling. Perhaps this would be a good time."	2
8. Reflect feeling	X	III	"You are explaining to me that your marital problems and job difficulties are not new experiences. How discouraging that must be."	2
9. Reflect meaning	X	III	"I am sorry, Darryl, that you are in such a desperate place in your life."	2
10. Clarifications	X			
11. Open-ended questions	X	IIII	"What do you want to do about all this, Darryl?"	2
12. Summarization	X	II	"I want to make sure I understand. Years ago, you remembered a time when your life was together. You enjoyed your single lifestyle, your dog, Alex, and your nursing job. Helping other people seemed the right thing to do. Is that accurate?"	2
13. Behavioral description	X	I	"From your voice and posture, you sound a bit ambivalent about being here."	2
14. Appropriate closed question	X	I	"It is okay that you go. We will see each other again. There are many ways of "going away," aren't there, Darryl?"	2
15. Perception check	X	I	"What ever is happening in your life is keeping you from having a healthy marriage and job. Sophia finds your work history unreliable, and Michael thinks you are angry some of the time. Is that correct?"	2
16. Silence	X	I	(I decided to be silent for at least 2 minutes!) "What were some of your saddest times, Darryl?"	2
17. Focusing	X	I	"Darryl, I appreciate your choosing, on some level, not to dissociate. That makes our work here easier. You will be okay in here. Let's focus again on a time when your life was not falling apart."	2
18. Feedback X		I	"There are those ambivalent feelings again, Darryl. Life has both happy and sad, doesn't it?"	2

Specific Criteria		Frequency	Comments	Skill Mastery Rating
C. Problem-solving skills/ defining skills				
1. Definition of Goals		I	"So you have at least two new coping skills to take with you to assist in the week to come. As a homework assignment for the next week, please share with Sophia what ever comes into your mind. I have a feeling she will appreciate sharing more than 'going away.' Also please spend at least 15 minutes a day with Michael doing some fun activity."	2
2. Exploration/understanding of concerns	X	II	"What do you hate about sad times, Darryl?"	2
3. Development/evaluation of alternatives	X	I	"You will shout again, but this time Michael will also have quality time to remember. Darryl, how committed are you to these two homework goals?"	2
4. Implement alternative				2
5. Special techniques		I	"You do not have to share them, Darryl."	2
6. Process counseling		I	"You and I have already started, Darryl. You will never be the same again, you have bravely faced the beast today in whatever form it appears."	2
D. Action phase/ confronting incongruities				
1. Immediacy				
2. Self-disclosure				
3. Confrontation				
4. Directives		I	"Help comes in many forms. If all your old ways of thinking and feelings have not worked, then let's try a different approach. Darryl, tell me the last time your life was not falling apart."	2
5. Logical consequences				
6. Interpretation		I	"My guess is that Sophia may be scared too and doesn't know what to do either."	2
E. Closing/generalization				
1. Summarization of content/feeling	X	I	"You applied your skills as a helping nurse practitioner to yourself! Wow! You shared and faced your fears. Darryl, when do you want to come back to counseling?"	2
2. Review of plan	X			
3. Rescheduling		I	"When do you want to come back to counseling?"	
4. Termination of session			2	
5. Evaluation of session	X	I	"You even coped differently here. Talk to me about how you coped differently today."	2
6. Follow-up				
F. Professionalism				
1. Developmental level match		I	"You are being very brave, Darryl. Tell me about your sad times."	2
2. Ethics				
3. Professional (punctual, attire, etc.)				

(*continued*)

RESOURCE S CONTINUED

Specific Criteria
G. Strengths: 1. Your micorcounseling skills were accomplished with intention and mastery. 2. You took your client's strengths as a medic and applied those skills to his current concerns.   Area for Improvement: 1. Be sure to deal with the multicultural issues as soon as your client is developmentally ready. 2. Continue to attend supervision sessions for added resources and assistance.   Total: 56

RESOURCE T

The Case of Darryl

(1) LORI: *Hi, Darryl, I am glad you came today.* (Greeting)

(2) DARRYL: *Me, too, I guess.*

(3) LORI: *From your voice and posture, you sound a bit ambivalent about being here.* (Behavioral description)

(4) DARRYL: *I do want to be here because I have so much to share, but I can't believe I was so scared that I began talking in tongues. I do that sometimes. My father was an evangelist. I am glad I didn't scare you off.*

(5) LORI: *You didn't scare me off. I know very little about talking in tongues. You will have to teach me more, but the two of us can make this a safe place to discuss anything you want. Last time I didn't take the time to explain how I do counseling. Perhaps this would be a good time.* (Verbal tracking; role definition)

(6) DARRYL: *Yes, I want to know more about the way you do counseling. So far, you are doing OK. You know, I have seen lots of other professionals, so I probably know the scoop. I like the fact you were sitting on the floor with me last time, though.*

(7) LORI: *I appreciate your giving me feedback, Darryl. As I will do the same with you. The more the two of us can become a team and build a counseling relationship, the better your counseling will go.* (Role definition/expectation)

(8) DARRYL: *You want me to work with you? Maybe I don't know the scoop, cuz most of the time people just tell me what to do.*

(9) LORI: *Darryl, I will not tell you what to do. My job is to listen to your concerns and assist you with your desired changes. I do not have the answers, but I can help you through the process of change.* (Role definition)

(10) DARRYL: *I thought you would have the answers!*

(11) LORI: *You have the answers, Darryl, to your problems. I can help you discover the needed answers by guiding you to the many possible solutions.* (Role definition)

(12) DARRYL: *I would like to find some solutions. I seem to have lots of problems.*

(13) LORI: *We all have problems, Darryl. Let's talk about your problems today, and by the end of this session, we will set several counseling goals to give us some counseling direction. How does that sound to you?* (Pacing; goal setting; open-ended question)

(14) DARRYL: *Strange, but good.*

(continued)

RESOURCE T CONTINUED

*(15) LORI: Darryl, what do you want to work on today in coun-
seling?* (Beginning)

*(16) DARRYL: My life seems to be falling apart. I am struggling in
my marriage, and I am having a difficult time keeping my job intact.
The most frustrating thing is that I have been in this place before.*

*(17) LORI: You are explaining to me that your marital problems
and job difficulties are not new experiences. How discouraging
that must be.* (Paraphrasing; reflection of feeling)

*(18) DARRYL: Yes, it is. It is deeper than discouragement, though,
this time it seems hopeless.*

*(19) LORI: I am sorry, Darryl, that you are in such a desperate
place in your life.* (Reflection of meaning)

*(20) DARRYL: Thanks for being so kind and understanding. My
wife, Sophia, thinks I am a bum. This is the third job I have had
since our marriage of 7 years. Our son, Michael, is 4, and he loves
to draw pictures. He drew a picture of me. I don't know exactly
what it means, but his depiction of me made me very sad. He drew
me shouting with a mouthful of teeth.*

*(21) LORI: What ever is happening in your life is keeping you
from having a healthy marriage and job. Sophia finds your work
history unreliable, and Michael thinks you are angry some of the
time. Is that correct?* (Paraphrase; perception check)

(22) DARRYL: Absolutely correct.

(23) LORI: What do you want to do about all this, Darryl? (Open-
ended question)

(24) DARRYL: I don't know. You are the counselor, you tell me.

*(25) LORI: It probably would be easier if I could tell you what to
do, but I can't, Darryl. Remember I don't have the answers to
your life.* (Focusing; role definition)

(26) DARRYL: Now you are not being helpful.

*(27) LORI: Help comes in many forms. If all your old ways of
thinking and feelings have not worked, then let's try a different
approach. Darryl, tell me the last time your life was not falling
apart.* (Directive)

*(28) DARRYL: (There is a long pause, and Darryl begins to stare. I
thought he might go into another trance-like, dissociative state.)*

*(29) LORI: Darryl, it is okay if you need to go away. I will be here
when you get back. You need to know that you are safe in here.*
(Empathy/rapport; respect)

*(30) DARRYL: (After several minutes of silence) I have been going
away for many years. Sophia hates it and screams at me.*

(31) LORI: *My guess is that Sophia may be scared too and doesn't know what to do either.* (Reflection of feeling; interpretation)

(32) DARRYL: *I think she just hates me because I am a no-good bum.*

(33) LORI: *Darryl, I appreciate your choosing, on some level, not to dissociate. That makes our work here easier. You will be okay in here. Let's focus again on a time when your life was not falling apart.* (Focusing)

(34) DARRYL: *Well, it was many years ago. I had decided that I would be single forever. I had my dog, Alex, and a good job as a nurse practitioner. My past was behind me. I felt good helping others and working in a doctor's office.*

(35) LORI: *I want to make sure I understand. Years ago, you remembered a time when your life was together. You enjoyed your single lifestyle, your dog, Alex, and your nursing job. Helping other people seemed the right thing to do. Is that accurate?* (Summarization; perception check)

(36) DARRYL: *Yes. Even hearing you talk about my old life makes me happy and sad.*

(37) LORI: *There are those ambivalent feelings again, Darryl. Life has both happy and sad, doesn't it?* (Feedback; verbal tracking)

(38) DARRYL: *Yes, but I hate sad times.*

(39) LORI: *What do you hate about sad times, Darryl?* (Open-ended question; exploration/understanding of concerns)

(40) DARRYL: *In my life there have been more sad times than not.*

(41) LORI: *(I decided to be silent for at least 2 minutes!) What were some of your saddest times, Darryl?* (Silence; open-ended questions; exploration)

(42) DARRYL: *(Tears were welling in his eyes.) My sad times are too sad to share!*

(43) LORI: *You do not have to share them, Darryl. (We sat in silence).* (Special technique—going with the resistance; rapport)

(44) DARRYL: *I want to share them with you, though.*

(45) LORI: *You are being very brave, Darryl. Tell me about your sad times.* (Feedback; directive; developmental match)

(46) DARRYL: *I was a medic in Viet Nam. I saw such devastation, but I honestly was doing okay. Knowing I was being helpful seemed to make the atrocities a little better. I helped many people, and I saw many men die.*

(47) LORI: *I can't imagine what you saw and lived through, but the fact that you saved so many people helped you through many difficult times.* (Reflection of meaning)

(48) DARRYL: *I guess so. One night my best friend, Stan, and I were together. Stan didn't have many friends and*

(continued)

RESOURCE T CONTINUED

he was kind of little. The other guys made fun of him. I really liked Stan. His friendship made the war more tolerable.

(49) LORI: Sounds as if you were a very good friend and that you helped people in many different ways. (Reflection of meaning)

(50) DARRYL: NO! I was not a good friend. I am done here. I need to go!

(51) LORI: Darryl, if you need to go, you can. Before you go, I want to give you an observation. When you were talking of Stan initially, your voice was soft and almost dreamy. When I suggested that you were a good friend to Stan, your voice became loud and aggressive. What are those voice changes about? (Feedback; behavioral description)

(52) DARRYL: I really need to go away.

(53) LORI: It is okay that you go. We will see each other again. There are many ways of "going away," aren't there, Darryl? (Rapport/empathy; closed question)

(54) DARRYL: You are really a pain in the neck.

(55) LORI: I can be a pain in the neck. I believe I am in good hands, though. (Verbal tracking)

(56) DARRYL: Okay, I won't go away, but you are not in good hands.

(57) LORI: You sound like a very competent nurse and friend, Darryl. Tell me why I am not in good hands. (Verbal tracking; directive)

(58) DARRYL: (Darryl begins shouting.) You are not in good hands, because these hands did not stop things I should have stopped. Are you happy now!

(59) LORI: I am not happy, Darryl, but I truly appreciate continuing to talk to me about such difficult times. (Feedback)

(60) DARRYL: I don't like to talk about my past. I haven't spoke a word of it to anyone, not even to my wife, Sophia.

(61) LORI: Then many memories are buried very deep. (Reflection of meaning)

(62) DARRYL: (Darryl begins to weep.)

(63) LORI: This must be very painful and devastating. (Reflection of feeling)

(64) DARRYL: It is more than devastating. It should not have happened. For years I wished I had been able to stop the hurt that we caused so many people.

(65) LORI: So for all these past years, you have carried around the burdens that you saw. (Paraphrase)

(66) DARRYL: Yes, I feel guilty for living. I have moments when I am happy with Sophia and Michael, but they are fleeting.

(67) LORI: *Tell me what you should have stopped.* (Directive)

(68) DARRYL: *One night, Stan and I were in a village and we heard sobbing and screaming. We approached the huts carefully and saw our own soldiers raping the village women. Stan and I told them to stop, but several of the men yelled at us to get lost and mind our own business. That night I went back to our temporary quarters, and I began having horrible nightmares! Those dreams still haunt me.*

(69) LORI: *That must have been frightening. And I would like to hear about your dreams, Darryl.* (Reflection of feeling; verbal tracking)

(70) DARRYL: *That is just it. I am not sure they were dreams.*

(71) LORI: *What do you mean you are not sure they were dreams?* (Open-ended question; exploration)

(72) DARRYL: *This is so difficult to say . . . I have been trying to piece together things.*

(73) LORI: *Tell me about those things, Darryl.* (Directive)

(74) DARRYL: *Well, I believe someone close to me sexually hurt me as a child. Bits and pieces come back to me, whether it be in dreams or vivid pictures in my head. I just don't know.*

(75) LORI: *There are so many of the dreams and pictures in your head that you believe they might be connected to a time when someone may have sexually hurt you. Is that right?* (Paraphrase; reflection of meaning)

(76) DARRYL: *I think so.*

(77) LORI: *Is it possible that the night in Viet Nam triggered some of your current behaviors and feelings?* (Interpretation)

(78) DARRYL: *I hadn't put the two together, but it makes some sense, as that is when the dreams began. I just don't want to believe that someone close could sexually harm me.*

(79) LORI: *You and I do not know if that is true or not. We may never know the truth, but that is not the issue here. Whether sexual abuse occurred or not is not the problem. We need to create a way for you to handle your present situation and your many perceptions about your past. Since we cannot change the past, one of our counseling goals is to change your perceptions of that past. That we can do.* (Goal setting; development/evaluation of alternatives)

(80) DARRYL: *That doesn't sound easy.*

(81) LORI: *It is not easy, but we can do it together as a team. How does that sound to you?* (Open-ended question)

(82) DARRYL: *Nothing else has been working, so it is worth a try. Where do we start?*

(83) LORI: *You and I have already started, Darryl. You will never be the same again, you have bravely faced the beast today in whatever form it appears.* (Feedback)

(continued)

(84) DARRYL: *It feels like such a long haul.*

(85) LORI: *It will be worth your effort, Darryl. The outcome may be that you learn new coping mechanisms to deal with your past and present.* (Goal setting)

(86) DARRYL: *I want my life to be different. I want Sophia and Michael to have a husband and father who can cope better with what ever life brings.*

(87) LORI: *I believe you can do that, Darryl. You even coped differently here. Talk to me about how you coped differently today.* (Feedback; directive)

(88) DARRYL: *(a long silence) I guess I did cope differently today. I felt strong enough to tell you things I have never shared . . . and I somehow did not "go away" when you asked me difficult questions.*

(89) LORI: *So you have at least two new coping skills to take with you to assist in the week to come. As a homework assignment for the next week, please share with Sophia what ever comes into your mind. I have a feeling she will appreciate sharing more than "going away." Also please spend at least 15 minutes a day with Michael doing some fun activity.* (Paraphrase; goal setting)

(90) DARRYL: *What if I shout at Michael again?*

(91) LORI: *You will shout again, but this time Michael will also have quality time to remember. Darryl, how committed are you to these two homework goals?* (Rapport; open-ended question)

(92) DARRYL: *I believe I can accomplish these two goals by sharing with Sophia and playing more with Michael.*

(93) LORI: *So you are committed to these goals. Before we go, I want to ask one more question. What kind of nurse were you in counseling today?* (Paraphrase; open-ended question; evaluation of session)

(94) DARRYL: *That is a funny question . . . but I guess I was a helpful and brave medic and nurse.*

(95) LORI: *You applied your skills as a helping nurse practitioner to yourself! Wow! You shared and faced your fears. Darryl, when do you want to come back to counseling?* (Summarization of content and feeling; rescheduling)

(96) DARRYL: *Do you have something available early in the week?*

(97) LORI: *There's an opening on Tuesday. See you at 10:00. Enjoy those competent nursing skills.* (Rapport; feedback, rescheduling)

Darryl and Lori continued to counsel together over a period of two years. During that time Darryl was hospitalized once for severe depression. Working conjointly with a psychiatrist, Darryl was placed on an antidepressant, and then continued in counseling with Lori. His prognosis was good, and he went back to work as a nurse practitioner.

WORKING WITH ETHICS, LAWS, AND PROFESSIONALISM: BEST PRACTICE STANDARDS

⇨ *Professional and ethical codes for the helping professions serve as guidelines defining good practice and standards of care.*

OVERVIEW

GOALS

KEY CONCEPTS: STANDARDS OF CARE

ETHICS AND ETHICAL BEHAVIORS
PRACTICAL REFLECTION 1: ETHICAL BEHAVIOR

CODE OF ETHICS
PRACTICAL REFLECTION 2: COMPREHENDING YOUR PROFESSION'S CODE OF ETHICS

CASE NOTES, RECORD KEEPING, AND HIPAA INFORMATION
PRACTICAL REFLECTION 3: WRITING CONCISE CASE NOTES FOCUSING ON HIPAA COMPLIANCE

THE PROCESS OF REFERRING CLIENTS TO OTHER PRACTITIONERS
PRACTICAL REFLECTION 4: THE REFERRAL PROCESS

UTILIZING CASE LAW
CONFIDENTIALITY AND DUTY TO WARN

EXCEPTIONS TO CONFIDENTIALITY
PRIVILEGED COMMUNICATION
PRACTICAL REFLECTION 5: UNDERSTANDING CASE LAW

PROFESSIONALISM AND PROFESSIONAL BEHAVIORS
PRACTICAL REFLECTION 6: RECOGNIZING PROFESSIONAL BEHAVIORS

PROFESSIONAL ORGANIZATIONS

ETHICAL AND PROFESSIONAL BEHAVIORS: THE CASE OF DARRYL
PRACTICAL REFLECTION 7: DILEMMAS IN THE CASE OF DARRYL

SUMMARY AND PERSONAL INTEGRATION
PRACTICAL REFLECTION 8: INTEGRATION

REFERENCES
RESOURCES U AND V

OVERVIEW

Students, faculty, and supervisors must be able to foster a sense of ethical behaviors and professionalism. Distinguishing these two elements and demonstrating appropriate behaviors is essential. Ethical guidelines for many of the helping professions will serve as resources. This chapter will also present landmark case law and the needed knowledge base to assist in decision making during the counseling process. Having a solid foundation about the origins of ethics, basic ethical guideline frameworks, and appropriate professional behavior will directly impact you and the way you practice in the helping professions. The newly mandated Health Insurance Portability and Accountability Act (HIPAA) requirements will also be introduced.

GOALS

1. Define and recognize ethical and professional behaviors.
2. Define and recognize issues of social justice.
3. Be aware of the ethical guidelines for helping professionals.
4. Understand the varying elements dictating ethical responsibility from codes and case law to professional organizations.
5. Identify specific case law that directly influences counseling decision making.
6. Comprehend the impact of the Health Insurance Portability and Accountability Act of 1996 (HIPAA) requirements on the helping professions.
7. Integrate the Case of Darryl into ethical and professional behaviors.

KEY CONCEPTS: STANDARDS OF CARE

When you go to any professional as a consumer of services, you expect a certain standard of care, whether it is a physician, lawyer, accountant, or other professional. You expect your chosen expert to have expertise and knowledge in the services you desire. You expect to be treated respectfully and competently. These are the same expectations for any consumer seeking out mental health services.

Embedded in these expectations is also the concept of social justice. Social justice as a standard of care is concerned with issues of human rights, fairness, and equity. Many clients will come to you having suffered from economic, racial/ethnic, gender-related, or other forms of oppression. Historically, counseling and therapy professions have not become directly involved in helping clients cope with cultural/environmental/contextual concerns. They have focused on individual counseling and therapy.

The National Association of Social Workers (1999) challenges this emphasis on the individual. They point out that many clients develop their problems because of external pressures of poverty, abuse, and prejudice. It is vital to help clients understand how their problems relate to their social context (Ivey & Ivey, 2003).

One ethical principle for social workers stipulates that social workers must challenge social injustice. Social workers pursue social change, particularly with a focus on working on behalf of vulnerable and oppressed individuals and groups. Social workers' social change efforts are focused primarily on issues of poverty, unemployment, discrimination, and other forms of social injustice. These activities seek to promote sensitivity to and knowledge about oppression and cultural and ethnic diversity. Social workers strive to ensure access to needed information, services, and resources; equality of opportunity and meaningful participation in decision making for all people (NASW, 1999).

Ethical practice:
Counseling behaviors that are guided by written organizational guidelines set forth through professional mandates.

The American Counseling Association (ACA) focuses the Preamble to its Code of Ethics on issues of diversity as an ethical matter. The ACA is an educational, scientific, and professional organization whose members are dedicated to the enhancement of human development throughout the lifespan. ACA members recognize diversity in our society and embrace a cross-cultural approach in support of the worth, dignity, potential, and uniqueness of each individual (ACA, 1995). The American Psychological Association (APA) also views diversity from an an ethical viewpoint (APA, 2002).

The Ethical Standards of Human Service Professionals (National Organization of Human Service Professionals, 2000) includes the following assertions:

Statement 17: Human service professionals provide services without discrimination or preference based on age, ethnicity, culture, race, disability, gender, religion, sexual orientation, or socioeconomic status.
Statement 18: Human service professionals are knowledgeable about the cultures and communities within which they practice. They are aware of multiculturalism in society and its impact on the community as well as individuals within the community. They respect individuals and groups, their cultures and beliefs.

As a helping professional, it is your counseling responsibility and duty to behave ethically, fairly, and professionally. These behaviors will be addressed throughout this chapter.

ETHICS AND ETHICAL BEHAVIORS

Ethical behaviors are guided by written organizational mandates adopted by a specific discipline. Later in this chapter you will have the opportunity to examine several codes of ethics. Examples of ethical behaviors that most of you easily recognize are clients' right to privacy, proper counseling relationships, and credentialing. These issues are written specifically in the ethical codes.

Authur and Swanson (1993) state,

> acting in an ethical manner can be summarized as emanating from six sources:
> - acts of the United States Congress or state legislation
> - common or case law
> - administrative law
> - professional association ethical standards
> - personal sociomoral values
> - state credentialing bodies providing licensure, certification, or registration which promulgate rules for practice and codes of ethics that become incorporated into law." (p. 6)

Confidentiality: The ethical duty to fulfill a contract or promise to clients that information gained through counseling will be protected from unauthorized disclosure (Authur & Swanson, 1993).

Informed consent: A client's rights to understand the limits and exceptions to confidentiality and the counseling relationship from the beginning of counseling.

Across the continuum of disciplines, the main features and functions of ethical guidelines seem to be similar and consistent. According to Koocher and Keith-Spiegel (1998), the related areas are promoting the dignity and welfare of your constituents; avoiding harm; establishing and maintaining your knowledge base and competence; ensuring confidentiality; avoiding dual relationships and conflicts of interest; and advocating for the integrity of your profession. Kaplan (2003) comments that 80% or more of all ethical concerns revolve around a single issue: informed consent. If that is the case, then it is essential that you have given your clients enough information about the counseling rules and expectations to decide whether or not to enter the therapeutic relationship. A verbal approach to informed consent is not enough. Refer back to the earlier example of informed consent. In this chapter you have several ethical guidelines to peruse. As you read the guidelines, you begin to notice that the standards do guide you, but they can never tell you the "right" way to make decision concerning clients.

We have discussed that ethical codes are designed to protect the consumer, but they also protect you as the practitioner and your profession (Baird, 2002). Three constructs that may guide you when making decisions about ethical dilemmas are autonomy, nonmaleficence, and beneficence (Beauchamp & Childress, 1995).

Autonomy suggests that your task as a helping professional is to assist your client in becoming independent as a person. *Nonmaleficence*

Practical Reflection 1: Ethical Behavior

Most ethical behaviors are derived from your organizational ethical codes. Select and discuss at least three ethical behaviors that you must demonstrate in your current placement site.

_____

_____

_____

_____

---

demands that you do no harm in any way to your client. *Beneficence* allows you to intervene in counseling to promote the good health, justice, and fidelity of your client's world. If you were to keep these three words in mind, it may assist you in making healthier ethical decisions.

CODE OF ETHICS

In most graduate courses you have taken in a mental health curricula, a professor has instructed you to read your discipline's professional organization Code of Ethics. Probably these same instructors have requested that you peruse the Code of Ethics from other professions as well. Many of these ethical guidelines are included in the resources at the end of this chapter, and each document has been written by members of that professional organization to assist you in providing quality treatment to your clients and to always do no harm (Baird, 2002).

You may view these codes and others on-line through the associations' homepages. Many web addresses are listed in Resource U. In addition there is a supplemental booklet available through this publisher entitled *Codes of Ethics for the Helping Professions* with codes from all helping professions' associations, such as the American Psychological Association, the National Association of Social Workers, and the National Organization for Human Service Education. You can purchase this 120-page booklet for approximately two dollars. Resource V displays the entire Code of Ethics from the American Counseling Association (ACA). Two additional sources of excellent ethical materials are Corey, Corey, and Callahan (2003) and Zuckerman (2003).

*Practical Reflection 2: Comprehending
Your Profession's Code of Ethics*

Read through the ethical guidelines in the resource section at the end of this chapter. How will these guidelines serve you during your field experience?

_____

_____

_____

_____

CASE NOTES, RECORD KEEPING, AND HIPAA INFORMATION

All ethical standards mention some aspect of keeping accurate counseling case notes; however, there seems to be a controversy surrounding exactly what should be included in the notes and where they can be stored. It is essential that you enter information from the counseling session into the record as soon as possible.

We like to write our case notes as soon as the client has left the appointment. That way the material is fresh in your mind. Date your entries, and try to be as concise as possible. This is not the place nor time to offer impressions, assumptions, or clichés about your client.

On some issues, particularly in the first interview, it may be wise to take notes during the session, but only if the client approves. One major advantage of a presession written history is that you do not have to take notes. Sometimes it is imperative to jot down notes. Try to remember what that may feel and look like to your client. We find that it usually distracts the client and does not help in building rapport. If you must take notes, let your client know that your notes are open records to that particular client and can be seen with you when requested. You could also tell your client what you have written. Sharing case notes with your clients can be an integral part of therapy.

Mitchell (1991) offers excellent examples of the need for clarity. A frequent goal may be, "Increase self-esteem," which is difficult to measure. A clearer version may be, "Will not be critical of self or personal decisions about disciplining children." Another example is, "Darryl is depressed." Again, how do we know Darryl is depressed? Mitchell suggests that we add a clarifying statement: "Darryl is depressed because he lost his job" (pp. 29–30).

It is also essential to focus on counseling goals for the client and list any session achievements and/or setbacks. Use behavioral and measurable terms. We have a standard form for case notes, which is attached to the intake form. Your own form or agency form might look something like this. Date: 6/10/2004 Goal: To introduce one new or old activity back into C.'s life. Demeanor: C. had shaved and was dressed in a clean and pressed company uniform. Outcome: C. did one random act of kindness for an anonymous person. Discussed stages of grief and loss.

Health Insurance Portability Account- ability Act: This 1996 Act requires helping professionals to ensure privacy and confidentiality of client information.

Remember these two helpful rules for writing case notes: Write as if your work is being subpoenaed for court, and always store your notes in a locked and safe file. Many codes of ethics stipulate these points, but they are also mandated by the new Health Insurance Portability and Accountability Act of 1996 (HIPAA). The U.S. Congress recognized the importance of protecting the privacy of patient and client health records, so uniform privacy standards were established. Privacy regulations include privacy, security, and electronic transmission standards. The HIPAA requires providers and others who maintain health information to design and implement security measures to safeguard the integrity and confidentiality of patient information (Tomes, 2001).

Agencies had until 2003 to comply with these privacy mandates. If an extension was filed, you may be exempt until October 16, 2003. The range of penalties for noncompliance may be from civil fines to criminal penalties. These are very serious regulations and persons or agencies in noncompliance may have fines up to $100 per person per violation or $250,000.00 and/or ten years' imprisonment, depending on the maliciousness of the crime. For many large companies, getting into compliance could be a costly and timely maneuver. For smaller counseling practices, compliance may be as simple as developing a security plan and/or locking client files. There are seven basic steps for developing and implementing a security system (Tomes, 2001).

1. Get management's commitment.
2. Appoint key personnel.
3. Perform a gap analysis of your agency's system for privacy.
4. Write and adopt a security policy and statement of information practices.
5. Perform a risk analysis of your agency methods and threats to confidentiality such as electronic records, and so on.
6. Implement security elements as necessary.
7. Test and revise your security system when needed.

For a thorough understanding of the HIPAA requirements, visit http://www.hhs.gov/ocr/hipaa. You could directly telephone the federal

Practical Reflection 3: Writing Concise Case Notes Focusing on HIPAA Compliance

Practice entering a short and valid case note. Be sure to make your goals measurable, describing behaviors not impressions. Describe where and how your case notes are stored. Share this information with your classmates.

_____

_____

_____

_____

Department of Health and Human Services (DHHS) for any questions concerning interpretation and application of the rules at 1-866-627-7748. The e-mail address for the DHHS is ocrprivacy@os.dhhs.gov. You may also inquire through your professional organization for updated information.

THE PROCESS OF REFERRING CLIENTS TO OTHER PRACTITIONERS

All ethical standards address the importance of referring clients when appropriate, and many guidelines stipulate that helping professionals must treat only those clients for whom they have qualified skills and competencies. Moursand and Kenny (2002) believe there are two basic questions that you must ask yourself when accepting or deciding to refer any client:

1. Will the client benefit from your services and area of expertise?
2. Do you and your client agree on similar counseling goals?

If the answer is yes to both these questions, then your decision to begin a counseling relationship has a solid foundation. Schuyler (1991) stated there are several aspects that create the necessary building blocks toward successful counseling outcomes. The client must want to seek help, have a readiness for change, and be open to communicating about personal concerns. The counselor must be able to instill a sense of hope, trust, and the need for commitment to the counseling process. The counselor must also be seen as confident, competent, and be able to create a

---

Practical Reflection 4: The Referral Process

Which clients, if any, have been assigned to your case load that you believe need to be referred? Ethically why should you refer them? Discuss.

_____

_____

_____

_____

---

counseling relationship that is warm and safe. If these conditions are not present, Schuyler believes a referral may be necessary.

UTILIZING CASE LAW

Case law: State and federal laws that set precedence for many helping professionals to follow.

In addition to utilizing the ethical codes, there are several landmark case laws that you need to understand to make solid ethical decisions; two will be presented. It is our hope that you will find these case laws interesting and challenging. Please continue to search out additional state and national case law that may assist you in your ethical decision making.

Confidentiality and Duty to Warn

Tarasoff v. Regents of the University of California 551 P.2d 334 (Cal. 1976) This suit occurred when Tatiana Tarasoff's parents sued their daughter's psychologist and the university with which he was affiliated for her wrongful death. Tatiana's boyfriend, Prosenjit Poddar, was the psychologist's patient. Mister Poddar revealed in a counseling session that he wanted to kill Tatiana when she returned home from a trip. Doctor Moore, the psychologist, felt that hospitalization was needed but he had to consult with others prior to such a decision. Poddar was examined by two additional psychiatrists, and a letter was sent to local police requesting their assistance in detaining Poddar. The police did interview Poddar, but by then he was denying his threats against Tatiana. Poddar was released. Two months later, Poddar attacked and killed Tatiana Tarasoff (CL 551 P.2d 334 Cal, 1976).

Exceptions to Confidentiality

1. Client is a danger to self and others.
2. Client requests the release of information and waives privacy.
3. A court orders the release of information.
4. Client gives up the right to confidentiality, when the counselor is receiving clinical supervision and client has been informed.
5. Client must be informed when office personnel will have access to billing and record keeping.
6. Client must be informed if legal and/or clinical consultation is needed.
7. Client raises the issue of their mental health in a legal proceeding.
8. A third party is present in the room.
9. Clients are under the age of 18. Check each state for age limit.
10. Client must be informed if informational sharing is a part of the treatment process.
11. Sharing of information is required in a penal system.
12. The client's purpose in disclosing information was to seek advice in the furtherance of a crime or fraud.
13. The counselor has reason to suspect child abuse.

Release of Information: A written contract by the client and a witness designating particular information that may be shared with stated professionals.

This case ruling of duty to warn has molded the very manner in which we explain confidentiality to our clients or patients. It is essential that you understand the importance of this ruling, the limits of confidentiality, and your duty to warn. The exceptions to confidentiality are numerous. Read about your duty to warn potential victims and proper authority when your client may be a danger to self or others, including drug use and criminal activity that has or may endanger human life. Authur and Swanson (1993) list thirteen total limits to confidentiality (pp. 19–20).

Maintaining confidentiality is your ethical counseling responsibility (Falvey, 2002). It is specifically written and delineated in every helping professions' Code of Ethics.

Privileged Communication

Jaffee v. Redmond 518 U.S. 1 (1996)   The case of *Jaffee v. Redmond* originated when a police officer shot and killed a man. The police officer entered into counseling with a licensed social worker. The deceased family brought about a federal civil suit against the police officer for wrongful death. During the trial the family's attorney requested the social worker's

Practical Reflection 5: Understanding Case Law

Describe how these case laws will be relevant to your field experiences and future counseling sessions.

_____

_____

_____

_____

Privileged communication: A client's legal right that confidences originating in a therapeutic relationship will be safeguarded during certain court proceedings (Authur & Swanson, 1993).

counseling case notes to see what comments had been made about the incident. The legal question arose whether there was "psychotherapist privilege" that would prevent the disclosure of the needed information (CL 518 U.S., 1996).

This Supreme Court decision has major implications for you as a helping professional. This landmark ruling establishes a new standard for privileged communication that prevents counseling communications from being shared in a court of law without written client or patient consent. For years only licensed psychiatrists and psychologists had psychotherapist privilege. After *Jaffe v. Redmond*, this privilege was expanded to include licensed psychotherapists in general, and all 50 states as well as the District of Columbia have passed into law some aspect of psychotherapist privilege (Falvey, 2002). In a computerized search of all U.S. jurisdictions, 98 percent of the jurisdictions that credentialed professional counselors showed evidence of granting privileged communications to the counselor–client relationship (Glosoff, Herlihy, & Spence, 2000). This holds true on a federal level, but it is up to you to locate and understand your state statutes.

PROFESSIONALISM AND PROFESSIONAL BEHAVIORS

How do ethical behaviors differ then from professional behaviors? Often we hear students say that certain behaviors are unethical. When encouraged to clarify the actions that are unethical, many times the behaviors are not unethical but unprofessional.

For example, where do you learn about the importance of punctuality and dressing appropriately for your counseling setting? We have been

---

Practical Reflection 6: Recognizing Professional Behaviors

Jot down several examples of professional behaviors that may be specific to your placement site. Discuss with your classmates.

_____

_____

_____

_____

Professionalism:
Counseling behaviors that are expected, although often are unwritten norms and cultures of agencies and disciplines.

taught in our ethical guidelines about confidentiality. Do our guidelines spell out specifically that we should not talk about clients with other counselors in elevators or over lunch? None of these behaviors are unethical; they are not spelled out in any ethical guidelines. However, they are critical, unprofessional, and related to the outcome of counseling.

Professional behaviors are dictated by your professional workplace and address job norms and expectations. Often professional behaviors are those that are spoken but unwritten norms of a particular agency or counseling culture, but you may find clarifications in workplace manuals and handbooks.

Be sure to check your agency handbooks for any rules and expectations that may be addressed in a policy manual. If these types of questions are not spelled out, please ask your supervisor or a colleague about special etiquette and/or professional behaviors. Remember that professionalism and the need for appropriate professional behaviors are as important as ethical behaviors. Be sure to discuss these professional behaviors with your supervisors. Adherence to these behaviors demonstrate standards of care for your clients, the profession, and you.

PROFESSIONAL ORGANIZATIONS

Another aspect of professionalism is belonging to a professional organization. Many of the same professors who requested that you read and understand the ethical guidelines may also encourage you to join a discipline-specific parent, division, and state organization. There are so many professional organizations for you to join, including the American Counseling Association (ACA), the American Mental Health Counseling Association (AMHCA), the American Psychological Association (APA), the National

Association for Social Workers (NASW), the Canadian Counseling Association, the Canadian Psychological Association, and the British Association for Counselling and Psychotherapy. These are parent organizations, and there are divisions within each of the above that emphasize inclusive concentrations, such as the American School Counselor Association (ASCA), the Association of Specialists in Group Work (ASGW), the Association for Multicultural Counseling and Development (AMCD), and many more.

The first, and perhaps the most important responsibility of membership, is a commitment to the profession. By becoming a member you are agreeing to abide by the organization's ethical guidelines. This commitment assists you in adhering to competency requirements of the discipline, but it also helps you in advocating for the needs of your clients and your discipline through your association's lobbying efforts. It was these same state, grassroots efforts that brought all the important licensing needs to the attention of your state legislature!

There are numerous other benefits to membership, such as refereed journals mailed to your home, library resources, insurance protection, and up-to-date information about the mental health profession. This information assists you in keeping informed, and learning about what your colleagues are practicing throughout the state, region, nation, and world. Consider joining through the mail or on-line—student membership rates are greatly reduced!

ETHICAL AND PROFESSIONAL BEHAVIORS: THE CASE OF DARRYL

As you review the Case of Darryl from Chapter 6, begin to think of the possible ethical and professional dilemmas that could occur. For example, when Darryl first goes into a dissociative state, did Lori have adequate skills to deal with Darryl? Is that an ethical and/or professional concern?

Another possible controversy concerns Lori's actions when she chose to sit on the floor with her client. Would that be considered an ethical and/or professional violation, if any? What are the potential privacy issues from HIPAA that need to be addressed?

SUMMARY AND PERSONAL INTEGRATION

The information in Chapter 7 defines your standards of care and offers good practice methods. Many ethical and professional issues were covered, but not everything you need to know about professional

Practical Reflection 7: Dilemmas in the Case of Darryl

Go over the script in the Case of Darryl. Write down any potential ethical and professional concerns that you observe. Also write any of Lori's behaviors that were ethical and professional. Share your ideas with your classmates.

_____

_____

_____

_____

Practical Reflection 8: Integration

After you review Chapter 7, outline the key ethical and professional issues that you would like to examine further. Discuss those with your classmates and supervisors.

_____

_____

_____

_____

and ethical decision making can be covered. Keep your Code of Ethics and agency manuals handy and continue to refer to them whenever you come across a professional and ethical dilemma.

In this chapter, you were introduced to guidelines and knowledge to assist you in becoming an ethical and professional mental health worker.

- Ethical and professional behaviors were defined and examples given.
- Sources and origins of ethical and professional practices were presented.
- Relevant landmark case laws were offered.
- HIPAA was introduced to assist in keeping client information confidential.
- The Case of Darryl was integrated into the chapter.

REFERENCES

American Counseling Association. (1995). American Counseling Association Code of Ethics and Standards of Practice. Alexandria, VA.

American Psychological Association. (2002). Ethical principles of psychologists and code of conduct. *American Psychologist, 46*, 1060–1073.

Authur, G. L., & Swanson, C. D. (1993). *The ACA Legal Series: Confidentiality and Privileged Communication*, vol. 6. Alexandria, VA: American Counseling Association.

Baird, B. N. (2002). *The Internship, Practicum, and Field Placement Handbook: A Guide for the Helping Professions* (3rd ed.). Upper Saddle River, NJ: Prentice Hall.

Beauchamp, T. L., & Childress, J. F. (1995). *Principles of Biomedical Ethics* (4th ed.). New York: Oxford University Press.

Corey, G., Corey, M., & Callanan, P. (2003). Issues and ethics in the helping professions. (6th ed.). Pacific Grove, CA: Brooks/Cole.

Glosoff, H. L., Herlihy, B., & Spence, E. B. (2000). Privileged communication in the counselor-client relationship. *Journal of Counseling & Development, 78*, 454–61.

Ivey, A., & Ivey, M. (2003). *Intentional Interviewing and Counseling: Facilitating Client Development in a Multicultural Society*. Pacific Grove, CA: Brooks/Cole.

Jaffee v. Redmond, 518 U.S. 1(1996).

Kaplan, D. (2003). Excellence in ethics. *Counseling Today*, 45/10, p.5.

Koocher, G., & Keith-Spiegel, P. (1998). *Ethics in Psychology: Professional Standards and Cases* (2nd ed). New York: Oxford University Press.

Mitchell, R. W. (1991). *The ACA Legal Series: Documentation in Counseling Records*, vol. 2, Alexandria, VA: American Counseling Association.

Moursand, J., & Kenny, M. (2002). *The Process of Counseling and Therapy* (4th ed.). Upper Saddle River, NJ: Prentice Hall.

National Association of Social Workers. (1999). *Code of Ethics*. Washington, DC.

National Organization of Human Service Professionals. (2000). Ethical standards of human service professionals. *Human Service Education, 20*, 61–8.

Schuyler, D. (1991). *A Practical Guide to Cognitive Therapy*. New York: W.W. Norton & Company.

Tarasoff v. Regents of the University of California, 551 P.2d 334 (Cal. 1976).

Tomes, J. T. (2001). *The Compliance Guide to HIPAA and the HHS Regulations*. Leawood, KS: Veterans Press.

Zuckerman, E. (2003). The paper office: Forms, guidelines, and resources to make your practice work ethically, legally and profitably. (3rd ed.). New York: Guildford Press.

RESOURCE U

Web Addresses for Professional Organizations and Codes of Ethics

American Association of Christian Counselors: Code of Ethics:
    http://www.aacc.net/code.html

American Association of Marriage and Family Therapy: Code of Ethics:
    http://www.aamft.org/about

American Association of Pastoral Counselors: Code of Ethics:
    http://www.agpc.org/ethics.html

American Counseling Association: Code of Ethics and Standards of
    Practice: http://www.counseling.org/resources/codeofethics.htm

American Group Psychotherapy Association: Guidelines for Ethics:
    http://www.groupsinc.org/group/ethicalguide.html

American Medical Association: Principles of Ethics:
    http://www.ama-assn.org

American Psychoanalytic Association: Principles and Standards of Ethics
    for Psychoanalysts: http://www.gpsa.org/ethics90l.html

American Psychological Association: Ethical Principles and Code of
    Conduct: http://www.apa.org/ethics/code.html

American School Counseling Association: Principles for Professional
    Ethics: http://www.schoolcounselor.org

Australian Psychological Society: Code of Ethics:
    http://www.psychsociety.com.au/about/finalcode.pdf

British Association for Counselling: Code of Ethics and Practice for
    Counsellors: http://bac.co.uk/members_visitors.htm

Canadian Counselling Association: Codes of Ethics:
    http://www.ccacc.ca/coe.htm

Canadian Psychological Association: http://www.cpa.ca

Commission on Rehabilitation Counselor Certification: Code of
    Professional Ethics: http://www.negia.net/~1234/ethics.html

Ethics Updates: http://ethics.acusd.edu

National Association of Alcoholism and Drug Abuse Counselors: Ethical
    Standards: http://naadac.org/ethics.htm

National Association of Social Workers: Code of Ethics:
    http://www.socialworkers.org/pubs/code/default.htm

National Board for Certified Counselors: Code of Ethics:
    http://www.nbcc.org/ethics/NBCCethics.htm

National Organization for Human Service Education: Ethical Standards:
    http://www.nohse.com/ethstand.html

New Zealand Association of Counsellors Inc.: Code of Ethics:
    http://www.nzac.org.nz/CodeOfEthics.html

RESOURCE V

ACA Code of Ethics and Standards of Practice*

ACA Code of Ethics
ACA Standards of Practice
References
Practitioner's Guide to Ethics
Frequently Asked Questions about Ethics
Policy And Procedures For Processing Complaints Of Ethical
    Violations
Layperson's Guide to Counselor Ethics
New: Ethical Standards for Internet Online Counseling

ACA Code of Ethics Preamble

The American Counseling Association is an educational, scientific, and professional organization whose members are dedicated to the enhancement of human development throughout the life-span. Association members recognize diversity in our society and embrace a cross-cultural approach in support of the worth, dignity, potential, and uniqueness of each individual.

   The specification of a code of ethics enables the association to clarify to current and future members, and to those served by members, the nature of the ethical responsibilities held in common by its members. As the code of ethics of the association, this document establishes principles that define the ethical behavior of association members. All members of the American Counseling Association are required to adhere to the Code of Ethics and the Standards of Practice. The Code of Ethics will serve as the basis for processing ethical complaints initiated against members of the association.

ACA Code of Ethics

Section A: The Counseling Relationship
Section B: Confidentiality
Section C: Professional Responsibility
Section D: Relationships With Other Professionals
Section E: Evaluation, Assessment, and Interpretation
Section F: Teaching, Training, and Supervision
Section G: Research and Publication
Section H: Resolving Ethical Issues

---

*Reprinted by permission of American Counseling Association.   *(continued)*

RESOURCE V CONTINUED

Section A: The Counseling Relationship

A.1. Client Welfare

   a. Primary Responsibility. The primary responsibility of counselors is to respect the dignity and to promote the welfare of clients.

   b. Positive Growth and Development. Counselors encourage client growth and development in ways that foster the clients' interest and welfare; counselors avoid fostering dependent counseling relationships.

   c. Counseling Plans. Counselors and their clients work jointly in devising integrated, individual counseling plans that offer reasonable promise of success and are consistent with abilities and circumstances of clients. Counselors and clients regularly review counseling plans to ensure their continued viability and effectiveness, respecting clients' freedom of choice. (See A.3.b.)

   d. Family Involvement. Counselors recognize that families are usually important in clients' lives and strive to enlist family understanding and involvement as a positive resource, when appropriate.

   e. Career and Employment Needs. Counselors work with their clients in considering employment in jobs and circumstances that are consistent with the clients' overall abilities, vocational limitations, physical restrictions, general temperament, interest and aptitude patterns, social skills, education, general qualifications, and other relevant characteristics and needs. Counselors neither place nor participate in placing clients in positions that will result in damaging the interest and the welfare of clients, employers, or the public.

A.2. Respecting Diversity

   a. Nondiscrimination. Counselors do not condone or engage in discrimination based on age, color, culture, disability, ethnic group, gender, race, religion, sexual orientation, marital status, or socioeconomic status. (See C.5.a., C.5.b., and D.1.i.)

   b. Respecting Differences. Counselors will actively attempt to understand the diverse cultural backgrounds of the clients with whom they work. This includes, but is not limited to, learning how the counselor's own cultural/ethnic/racial identity impacts her or his values and beliefs about the counseling process. (See E.8. and F.2.i.)

A.3. Client Rights

   a. Disclosure to Clients. When counseling is initiated, and throughout the counseling process as necessary, counselors inform clients of the purposes, goals, techniques, procedures, limitations, potential risks, and benefits of services to be performed, and other pertinent information. Counselors take steps to ensure that clients understand the implications of diagnosis, the intended use of tests and reports, fees, and billing arrangements. Clients have the right to expect confidentiality and to be provided with an explanation of its limitations, including supervision and/or treatment team professionals; to obtain clear information about their case records; to participate in the ongoing counseling plans; and to refuse any recommended services and be advised of the consequences of such refusal. (See E.5.a. and G.2.)

b. Freedom of Choice. Counselors offer clients the freedom to choose whether to enter into a counseling relationship and to determine which professional(s) will provide counseling. Restrictions that limit choices of clients are fully explained. (See A.1.c.)

c. Inability to Give Consent. When counseling minors or persons unable to give voluntary informed consent, counselors act in these clients' best interests. (See B.3.)

A.4. Clients Served by Others

If a client is receiving services from another mental health professional, counselors, with client consent, inform the professional persons already involved and develop clear agreements to avoid confusion and conflict for the client. (See C.6.c.)

A.5. Personal Needs and Values

a. Personal Needs. In the counseling relationship, counselors are aware of the intimacy and responsibilities inherent in the counseling relationship, maintain respect for clients, and avoid actions that seek to meet their personal needs at the expense of clients.

b. Personal Values. Counselors are aware of their own values, attitudes, beliefs, and behaviors and how these apply in a diverse society, and avoid imposing their values on clients. (See C.5.a.)

A.6. Dual Relationships

a. Avoid When Possible. Counselors are aware of their influential positions with respect to clients, and they avoid exploiting the trust and dependency of clients. Counselors make every effort to avoid dual relationships with clients that could impair professional judgment or increase the risk of harm to clients. (Examples of such relationships include, but are not limited to, familial, social, financial, business, or close personal relationships with clients.) When a dual relationship cannot be avoided, counselors take appropriate professional precautions such as informed consent, consultation, supervision, and documentation to ensure that judgment is not impaired and no exploitation occurs. (See F.1.b.)

(continued)

RESOURCE V CONTINUED

b. Superior/Subordinate Relationships. Counselors do not accept as clients superiors or subordinates with whom they have administrative, supervisory, or evaluative relationships.

A.7. Sexual Intimacies With Clients

a. Current Clients. Counselors do not have any type of sexual intimacies with clients and do not counsel persons with whom they have had a sexual relationship.

b. Former Clients. Counselors do not engage in sexual intimacies with former clients within a minimum of 2 years after terminating the counseling relationship. Counselors who engage in such relationship after 2 years following termination have the responsibility to examine and document thoroughly that such relations did not have an exploitative nature, based on factors such as duration of counseling, amount of time since counseling, termination circumstances, client's personal history and mental status, adverse impact on the client, and actions by the counselor suggesting a plan to initiate a sexual relationship with the client after termination.

A.8. Multiple Clients

When counselors agree to provide counseling services to two or more persons who have a relationship (such as husband and wife, or parents and children), counselors clarify at the outset which person or persons are clients and the nature of the relationships they will have with each involved person. If it becomes apparent that counselors may be called upon to perform potentially conflicting roles, they clarify, adjust, or withdraw from roles appropriately. (See B.2. and B.4.d.)

A.9. Group Work

a. Screening. Counselors screen prospective group counseling/therapy participants. To the extent possible, counselors select members whose needs and goals are compatible with goals of the group, who will not impede the group process, and whose well-being will not be jeopardized by the group experience.

b. Protecting Clients. In a group setting, counselors take reasonable precautions to protect clients from physical or psychological trauma.

A.10. Fees and Bartering (See D.3.a. and D.3.b.)

a. Advance Understanding. Counselors clearly explain to clients, prior to entering the counseling relationship, all financial arrangements related to professional services including the use of collection agencies or legal measures for nonpayment. (A.11.c.)

b. Establishing Fees. In establishing fees for professional counseling services, counselors consider the financial status of clients and locality. In the event that the established fee structure is inappropriate for a client, assistance is provided in attempting to find comparable services of acceptable cost. (See A.10.d., D.3.a., and D.3.b.)

c. Bartering Discouraged. Counselors ordinarily refrain from accepting goods or services from clients in return for counseling services because such arrangements create inherent potential for conflicts, exploitation, and distortion of the professional relationship. Counselors may participate in bartering only if the relationship is not exploitative, if the client requests it, if a clear written contract is established, and if such arrangements are an accepted practice among professionals in the community. (See A.6.a.)

d. Pro Bono Service. Counselors contribute to society by devoting a portion of their professional activity to services for which there is little or no financial return (pro bono).

A.11. Termination and Referral

a. Abandonment Prohibited. Counselors do not abandon or neglect clients in counseling. Counselors assist in making appropriate arrangements for the continuation of treatment, when necessary, during interruptions such as vacations, and following termination.

b. Inability to Assist Clients. If counselors determine an inability to be of professional assistance to clients, they avoid entering or immediately terminate a counseling relationship. Counselors are knowledgeable about referral resources and suggest appropriate alternatives. If clients decline the suggested referral, counselors should discontinue the relationship.

c. Appropriate Termination. Counselors terminate a counseling relationship, securing client agreement when possible, when it is reasonably clear that the client is no longer benefiting, when services are no longer required, when counseling no longer serves the client's needs or interests, when clients do not pay fees charged, or when agency or institution limits do not allow provision of further counseling services. (See A.10.b. and C.2.g.)

A.12. Computer Technology

a. Use of Computers. When computer applications are used in counseling services, counselors ensure that (1) the client is intellectually, emotionally, and physically capable of using the computer application; (2) the computer application is appropriate for the needs of the client; (3) the client understands the purpose and operation of the computer applications; and (4) a follow-up of client use of a computer application is provided to correct possible misconceptions, discover inappropriate use, and assess subsequent needs.

(continued)

RESOURCE V CONTINUED

b. Explanation of Limitations. Counselors ensure that clients are provided information as a part of the counseling relationship that adequately explains the limitations of computer technology.

c. Access to Computer Applications. Counselors provide for equal access to computer applications in counseling services. (See A.2.a.)

Section B: Confidentiality

B.1. Right to Privacy

a. Respect for Privacy. Counselors respect their clients right to privacy and avoid illegal and unwarranted disclosures of confidential information. (See A.3.a. and B.6.a.)

b. Client Waiver. The right to privacy may be waived by the client or his or her legally recognized representative.

c. Exceptions. The general requirement that counselors keep information confidential does not apply when disclosure is required to prevent clear and imminent danger to the client or others or when legal requirements demand that confidential information be revealed. Counselors consult with other professionals when in doubt as to the validity of an exception.

d. Contagious, Fatal Diseases. A counselor who receives information confirming that a client has a disease commonly known to be both communicable and fatal is justified in disclosing information to an identifiable third party, who by his or her relationship with the client is at a high risk of contracting the disease. Prior to making a disclosure the counselor should ascertain that the client has not already informed the third party about his or her disease and that the client is not intending to inform the third party in the immediate future. (See B.1.c and B.1.f.)

e. Court-Ordered Disclosure. When court ordered to release confidential information without a client's permission, counselors request to the court that the disclosure not be required due to potential harm to the client or counseling relationship. (See B.1.c.)

f. Minimal Disclosure. When circumstances require the disclosure of confidential information, only essential information is revealed. To the extent possible, clients are informed before confidential information is disclosed.

g. Explanation of Limitations. When counseling is initiated and throughout the counseling process as necessary, counselors inform clients of the limitations of confidentiality and identify foreseeable situations in which confidentiality must be breached. (See G.2.a.)

h. Subordinates. Counselors make every effort to ensure that privacy and confidentiality of clients are maintained by subordinates including employees, supervisees, clerical assistants, and volunteers. (See B.1.a.)

i. Treatment Teams. If client treatment will involve a continued review by a treatment team, the client will be informed of the team's existence and composition.

B.2. Groups and Families

a. Group Work. In group work, counselors clearly define confidentiality and the parameters for the specific group being entered, explain its importance, and discuss the difficulties related to confidentiality involved in group work. The fact that confidentiality cannot be guaranteed is clearly communicated to group members.

b. Family Counseling. In family counseling, information about one family member cannot be disclosed to another member without permission. Counselors protect the privacy rights of each family member. (See A.8., B.3., and B.4.d.)

B.3. Minor or Incompetent Clients

When counseling clients who are minors or individuals who are unable to give voluntary, informed consent, parents or guardians may be included in the counseling process as appropriate. Counselors act in the best interests of clients and take measures to safeguard confidentiality. (See A.3.c.)

B.4. Records

a. Requirement of Records. Counselors maintain records necessary for rendering professional services to their clients and as required by laws, regulations, or agency or institution procedures.

b. Confidentiality of Records. Counselors are responsible for securing the safety and confidentiality of any counseling records they create, maintain, transfer, or destroy whether the records are written, taped, computerized, or stored in any other medium. (See B.1.a.)

c. Permission to Record or Observe. Counselors obtain permission from clients prior to electronically recording or observing sessions. (See A.3.a.)

d. Client Access. Counselors recognize that counseling records are kept for the benefit of clients, and therefore provide access to records and copies of records when requested by competent clients, unless the records contain information that may be misleading and detrimental to the client. In situations involving multiple clients, access to records is limited to those parts of records that do not include confidential information related to another client. (See A.8., B.1.a., and B.2.b.)

(continued)

RESOURCE V CONTINUED

e. Disclosure or Transfer. Counselors obtain written permission from clients to disclose or transfer records to legitimate third parties unless exceptions to confidentiality exist as listed in Section B.1. Steps are taken to ensure that receivers of counseling records are sensitive to their confidential nature.

B.5. Research and Training

a. Data Disguise Required. Use of data derived from counseling relationships for purposes of training, research, or publication is confined to content that is disguised to ensure the anonymity of the individuals involved. (See B.1.g. and G.3.d.)

b. Agreement for Identification. Identification of a client in a presentation or publication is permissible only when the client has reviewed the material and has\ agreed to its presentation or publication. (See G.3.d.)

B.6. Consultation

a. Respect for Privacy. Information obtained in a consulting relationship is discussed for professional purposes only with persons clearly concerned with the case. Written and oral reports present data germane to the purposes of the consultation, and every effort is made to protect client identity and avoid undue invasion of privacy.

b. Cooperating Agencies. Before sharing information, counselors make efforts to ensure that there are defined policies in other agencies serving the counselor's clients that effectively protect the confidentiality of information.

Section C: Professional Responsibility

C.1. Standards Knowledge

Counselors have a responsibility to read, understand, and follow the Code of Ethics and the Standards of Practice.

C.2. Professional Competence

a. Boundaries of Competence. Counselors practice only within the boundaries of their competence, based on their education, training, supervised experience, state and national professional credentials, and appropriate professional experience. Counselors will demonstrate a commitment to gain knowledge, personal awareness, sensitivity, and skills pertinent to working with a diverse client population.

b. New Specialty Areas of Practice. Counselors practice in specialty areas new to them only after appropriate education, training, and supervised experience. While developing skills in new specialty areas, counselors take steps to ensure the competence of their work and to protect others from possible harm.

    c. Qualified for Employment. Counselors accept employment only for positions for which they are qualified by education, training, supervised experience, state and national professional credentials, and appropriate professional experience. Counselors hire for professional counseling positions only individuals who are qualified and competent.

    d. Monitor Effectiveness. Counselors continually monitor their effectiveness as professionals and take steps to improve when necessary. Counselors in private practice take reasonable steps to seek out peer supervision to evaluate their efficacy as counselors.

    e. Ethical Issues Consultation. Counselors take reasonable steps to consult with other counselors or related professionals when they have questions regarding their ethical obligations or professional practice. (See H.1.)

    f. Continuing Education. Counselors recognize the need for continuing education to maintain a reasonable level of awareness of current scientific and professional information in their fields of activity. They take steps to maintain competence in the skills they use, are open to new procedures, and keep current with the diverse and/or special populations with whom they work.

    g. Impairment. Counselors refrain from offering or accepting professional services when their physical, mental, or emotional problems are likely to harm a client or others. They are alert to the signs of impairment, seek assistance for problems, and, if necessary, limit, suspend, or terminate their professional responsibilities. (See A.11.c.)

C.3. Advertising and Soliciting Clients

    a. Accurate Advertising. There are no restrictions on advertising by counselors except those that can be specifically justified to protect the public from deceptive practices. Counselors advertise or represent their services to the public by identifying their credentials in an accurate manner that is not false, misleading, deceptive, or fraudulent. Counselors may only advertise the highest degree earned which is in counseling or a closely related field from a college or university that was accredited when the degree was awarded by one of the regional accrediting bodies recognized by the Council on Postsecondary Accreditation.

    b. Testimonials. Counselors who use testimonials do not solicit them from clients or other persons who, because of their particular circumstances, may be vulnerable to undue influence.

    c. Statements by Others. Counselors make reasonable efforts to ensure that statements made by others about them or the profession of counseling are accurate.

(continued)

RESOURCE V CONTINUED

d. Recruiting Through Employment. Counselors do not use their places of employment or institutional affiliation to recruit or gain clients, supervisees, or consultees for their private practices. (See C.5.e.)

e. Products and Training Advertisements. Counselors who develop products related to their profession or conduct workshops or training events ensure that the advertisements concerning these products or events are accurate and disclose adequate information for consumers to make informed choices.

f. Promoting to Those Served. Counselors do not use counseling, teaching, training, or supervisory relationships to promote their products or training events in a manner that is deceptive or would exert undue influence on individuals who may be vulnerable. Counselors may adopt textbooks they have authored for instruction purposes.

g. Professional Association Involvement. Counselors actively participate in local, state, and national associations that foster the development and improvement of counseling.

C.4. Credentials

a. Credentials Claimed. Counselors claim or imply only professional credentials possessed and are responsible for correcting any known misrepresentations of their credentials by others. Professional credentials include graduate degrees in counseling or closely related mental health fields, accreditation of graduate programs, national voluntary certifications, government-issued certifications or licenses, ACA professional membership, or any other credential that might indicate to the public specialized knowledge or expertise in counseling.

b. ACA Professional Membership. ACA professional members may announce to the public their membership status. Regular members may not announce their ACA membership in a manner that might imply they are credentialed counselors.

c. Credential Guidelines. Counselors follow the guidelines for use of credentials that have been established by the entities that issue the credentials.

d. Misrepresentation of Credentials. Counselors do not attribute more to their credentials than the credentials represent, and do not imply that other counselors are not qualified because they do not possess certain credentials.

e. Doctoral Degrees From Other Fields. Counselors who hold a master's degree in counseling or a closely related mental health field, but hold a doctoral degree from other than counseling or a closely related field, do not use the title "Dr." in their practices and do not announce to the public in relation to their practice or status as a counselor that they hold a doctorate.

C.5. Public Responsibility

a. Nondiscrimination. Counselors do not discriminate against clients, students, or supervisees in a manner that has a negative impact based on their age, color, culture, disability, ethnic group, gender, race, religion, sexual orientation, or socioeconomic status, or for any other reason. (See A.2.a.)

b. Sexual Harassment. Counselors do not engage in sexual harassment. Sexual harassment is defined as sexual solicitation, physical advances, or verbal or nonverbal conduct that is sexual in nature, that occurs in connection with professional activities or roles, and that either (1) is unwelcome, is offensive, or creates a hostile workplace environment, and counselors know or are told this; or (2) is sufficiently severe or intense to be perceived as harassment to a reasonable person in the context. Sexual harassment can consist of a single intense or severe act or multiple persistent or pervasive acts.

c. Reports to Third Parties. Counselors are accurate, honest, and unbiased in reporting their professional activities and judgments to appropriate third parties including courts, health insurance companies, those who are the recipients of evaluation reports, and others. (See B.1.g.)

d. Media Presentations. When counselors provide advice or comment by means of public lectures, demonstrations, radio or television programs, prerecorded tapes, printed articles, mailed material, or other media, they take reasonable precautions to ensure that (1) the statements are based on appropriate professional counseling literature and practice; (2) the statements are otherwise consistent with the Code of Ethics and the Standards of Practice; and (3) the recipients of the information are not encouraged to infer that a professional counseling relationship has been established. (See C.6.b.)

e. Unjustified Gains. Counselors do not use their professional positions to seek or receive unjustified personal gains, sexual favors, unfair advantage, or unearned goods or services. (See C.3.d.)

C.6. Responsibility to Other Professionals

a. Different Approaches. Counselors are respectful of approaches to professional counseling that differ from their own. Counselors know and take into account the traditions and practices of other professional groups with which they work.

b. Personal Public Statements. When making personal statements in a public context, counselors clarify that they are speaking

(continued)

RESOURCE V CONTINUED

from their personal perspectives and that they are not speaking on behalf of all counselors or the profession. (See C.5.d.)

c. Clients Served by Others. When counselors learn that their clients are in a professional relationship with another mental health professional, they request release from clients to inform the other professionals and strive to establish positive and collaborative professional relationships. (See A.4.)

Section D: Relationships With Other Professionals

D.1. Relationships With Employers and Employees

a. Role Definition. Counselors define and describe for their employers and employees the parameters and levels of their professional roles.

b. Agreements. Counselors establish working agreements with supervisors, colleagues, and subordinates regarding counseling or clinical relationships, confidentiality, adherence to professional standards, distinction between public and private material, maintenance and dissemination of recorded information, work load, and accountability. Working agreements in each instance are specified and made known to those concerned.

c. Negative Conditions. Counselors alert their employers to conditions that may be potentially disruptive or damaging to the counselor's professional responsibilities or that may limit their effectiveness.

d. Evaluation. Counselors submit regularly to professional review and evaluation by their supervisor or the appropriate representative of the employer.

e. In-Service. Counselors are responsible for in-service development of self and staff.

f. Goals. Counselors inform their staff of goals and programs.

g. Practices. Counselors provide personnel and agency practices that respect and enhance the rights and welfare of each employee and recipient of agency services. Counselors strive to maintain the highest levels of professional services.

h. Personnel Selection and Assignment. Counselors select competent staff and assign responsibilities compatible with their skills and experiences.

i. Discrimination. Counselors, as either employers or employees, do not engage in or condone practices that are inhumane, illegal, or unjustifiable (such as considerations based on age, color, culture, disability, ethnic group, gender, race, religion, sexual orientation, or socioeconomic status) in hiring, promotion, or training. (See A.2.a. and C.5.b.)

    j. Professional Conduct. Counselors have a responsibility both to clients and to the agency or institution within which services are performed to maintain high standards of professional conduct.

    k. Exploitative Relationships. Counselors do not engage in exploitative relationships with individuals over whom they have supervisory, evaluative, or instructional control or authority.

    l. Employer Policies. The acceptance of employment in an agency or institution implies that counselors are in agreement with its general policies and principles. Counselors strive to reach agreement with employers as to acceptable standards of conduct that allow for changes in institutional policy conducive to the growth and development of clients.

D.2. Consultation (See B.6.)

    a. Consultation as an Option. Counselors may choose to consult with any other professionally competent persons about their clients. In choosing consultants, counselors avoid placing the consultant in a conflict of interest situation that would preclude the consultant being a proper party to the counselor's efforts to help the client. Should counselors be engaged in a work setting that compromises this consultation standard, they consult with other professionals whenever possible to consider justifiable alternatives.

    b. Consultant Competency. Counselors are reasonably certain that they have or the organization represented has the necessary competencies and resources for giving the kind of consulting services needed and that appropriate referral resources are available.

    c. Understanding With Clients. When providing consultation, counselors attempt to develop with their clients a clear understanding of problem definition, goals for change, and predicted consequences of interventions selected.

    d. Consultant Goals. The consulting relationship is one in which client adaptability and growth toward self-direction are consistently encouraged and cultivated. (See A.1.b.)

D.3. Fees for Referral

    a. Accepting Fees From Agency Clients. Counselors refuse a private fee or other remuneration for rendering services to persons who are entitled to such services through the counselor's employing agency or institution. The policies of a particular agency may make explicit provisions for agency clients to receive counseling services from members of its staff in private practice. In such instances, the clients must be informed of other options open to them should they seek private counseling services. (See A.10.a., A.11.b., and C.3.d.)

    b. Referral Fees. Counselors do not accept a referral fee from other professionals.

(continued)

RESOURCE V CONTINUED

D.4.   Subcontractor Arrangements
When counselors work as subcontractors for counseling services for a third party, they have a duty to inform clients of the limitations of confidentiality that the organization may place on counselors in providing counseling services to clients. The limits of such confidentiality ordinarily are discussed as part of the intake session. (See B.1.e. and B.1.f.)

Section E: Evaluation, Assessment, and Interpretation

E.1.   General
   a. Appraisal Techniques. The primary purpose of educational and psychological assessment is to provide measures that are objective and interpretable in either comparative or absolute terms. Counselors recognize the need to interpret the statements in this section as applying to the whole range of appraisal techniques, including test and nontest data.
   b. Client Welfare. Counselors promote the welfare and best interests of the client in the development, publication, and utilization of educational and psychological assessment techniques. They do not misuse assessment results and interpretations and take reasonable steps to prevent others from misusing the information these techniques provide. They respect the client's right to know the results, the interpretations made, and the bases for their conclusions and recommendations.

E.2.   Competence to Use and Interpret Tests
   a. Limits of Competence. Counselors recognize the limits of their competence and perform only those testing and assessment services for which they have been trained. They are familiar with reliability, validity, related standardization, error of measurement, and proper application of any technique utilized. Counselors using computer-based test interpretations are trained in the construct being measured and the specific instrument being used prior to using this type of computer application. Counselors take reasonable measures to ensure the proper use of psychological assessment techniques by persons under their supervision.
   b. Appropriate Use. Counselors are responsible for the appropriate application, scoring, interpretation, and use of assessment instruments, whether they score and interpret such tests themselves or use computerized or other services.
   c. Decisions Based on Results. Counselors responsible for decisions involving individuals or policies that are based on assessment results have a thorough understanding of educational and

        psychological measurement, including validation criteria, test
research, and guidelines for test development and use.

    d. Accurate Information. Counselors provide accurate information
and avoid false claims or misconceptions when making statements about assessment instruments or techniques. Special efforts are made to avoid unwarranted connotations of such terms as IQ and grade equivalent scores. (See C.5.c.)

E.3. Informed Consent

    a. Explanation to Clients. Prior to assessment, counselors explain
the nature and purposes of assessment and the specific use of results in language the client (or other legally authorized person on behalf of the client) can understand, unless an explicit exception to this right has been agreed upon in advance. Regardless of whether scoring and interpretation are completed by counselors, by assistants, or by computer or other outside services, counselors take reasonable steps to ensure that appropriate explanations are given to the client.

    b. Recipients of Results. The examinee's welfare, explicit understanding, and prior agreement determine the recipients of test results. Counselors include accurate and appropriate interpretations with any release of individual or group test results. (See B.1.a. and C.5.c.)

E.4. Release of Information to Competent Professionals

    a. Misuse of Results. Counselors do not misuse assessment results, including test results, and interpretations, and take reasonable steps to prevent the misuse of such by others. (See C.5.c.)

    b. Release of Raw Data. Counselors ordinarily release data (e.g., protocols, counseling or interview notes, or questionnaires) in which the client is identified only with the consent of the client or the client's legal representative. Such data are usually released only to persons recognized by counselors as competent to interpret the data. (See B.1.a.)

E.5. Proper Diagnosis of Mental Disorders

    a. Proper Diagnosis. Counselors take special care to provide proper diagnosis of mental disorders. Assessment techniques (including personal interview) used to determine client care (e.g., locus of treatment, type of treatment, or recommended follow-up) are carefully selected and appropriately used. (See A.3.a. and C.5.c.)

    b. Cultural Sensitivity. Counselors recognize that culture affects the manner in which clients' problems are defined. Clients' socioeconomic and cultural experience is considered when diagnosing mental disorders.

(continued)

RESOURCE V CONTINUED

E.6. Test Selection
- a. Appropriateness of Instruments. Counselors carefully consider the validity, reliability, psychometric limitations, and appropriateness of instruments when selecting tests for use in a given situation or with a particular client.
- b. Culturally Diverse Populations. Counselors are cautious when selecting tests for culturally diverse populations to avoid inappropriateness of testing that may be outside of socialized behavioral or cognitive patterns.

E.7. Conditions of Test Administration
- a. Administration Conditions. Counselors administer tests under the same conditions that were established in their standardization. When tests are not administered under standard conditions or when unusual behavior or irregularities occur during the testing session, those conditions are noted in interpretation, and the results may be designated as invalid or of questionable validity.
- b. Computer Administration. Counselors are responsible for ensuring that administration programs function properly to provide clients with accurate results when a computer or other electronic methods are used for test administration. (See A.12.b.)
- c. Unsupervised Test Taking. Counselors do not permit unsupervised or inadequately supervised use of tests or assessments unless the tests or assessments are designed, intended, and validated for self-administration and/or scoring.
- d. Disclosure of Favorable Conditions. Prior to test administration, conditions that produce most favorable test results are made known to the examinee.

E.8. Diversity in Testing
Counselors are cautious in using assessment techniques, making evaluations, and interpreting the performance of populations not represented in the norm group on which an instrument was standardized. They recognize the effects of age, color, culture, disability, ethnic group, gender, race, religion, sexual orientation, and socioeconomic status on test administration and interpretation and place test results in proper perspective with other relevant factors. (See A.2.a.)

E.9. Test Scoring and Interpretation
- a. Reporting Reservations. In reporting assessment results, counselors indicate any reservations that exist regarding validity or reliability because of the circumstances of the assessment or the inappropriateness of the norms for the person tested.

b. Research Instruments. Counselors exercise caution when interpreting the results of research instruments possessing insufficient technical data to support respondent results. The specific purposes for the use of such instruments are stated explicitly to the examinee.

c. Testing Services. Counselors who provide test scoring and test interpretation services to support the assessment process confirm the validity of such interpretations. They accurately describe the purpose, norms, validity, reliability, and applications of the procedures and any special qualifications applicable to their use. The public offering of an automated test interpretations service is considered a professional-to-professional consultation. The formal responsibility of the consultant is to the consultee, but the ultimate and overriding responsibility is to the client.

E.10. Test Security

Counselors maintain the integrity and security of tests and other assessment techniques consistent with legal and contractual obligations. Counselors do not appropriate, reproduce, or modify published tests or parts thereof without acknowledgment and permission from the publisher.

E.11. Obsolete Tests and Outdated Test Results

Counselors do not use data or test results that are obsolete or outdated for the current purpose. Counselors make every effort to prevent the misuse of obsolete measures and test data by others.

E.12. Test Construction

Counselors use established scientific procedures, relevant standards, and current professional knowledge for test design in the development, publication, and utilization of educational and psychological assessment techniques.

Section F: Teaching, Training, and Supervision

F.1. Counselor Educators and Trainers

a. Educators as Teachers and Practitioners. Counselors who are responsible for developing, implementing, and supervising educational programs are skilled as teachers and practitioners. They are knowledgeable regarding the ethical, legal, and regulatory aspects of the profession, are skilled in applying that knowledge, and make students and supervisees aware of their responsibilities. Counselors conduct counselor education and training programs in an ethical manner and serve as role models for professional behavior. Counselor educators should make an effort to infuse material related to human diversity into all courses and/or workshops that are designed to promote the development of professional counselors.

(continued)

RESOURCE V CONTINUED

b. Relationship Boundaries With Students and Supervisees. Counselors clearly define and maintain ethical, professional, and social relationship boundaries with their students and supervisees. They are aware of the differential in power that exists and the student's or supervisee's possible incomprehension of that power differential. Counselors explain to students and supervisees the potential for the relationship to become exploitive.

c. Sexual Relationships. Counselors do not engage in sexual relationships with students or supervisees and do not subject them to sexual harassment. (See A.6. and C.5.b)

d. Contributions to Research. Counselors give credit to students or supervisees for their contributions to research and scholarly projects. Credit is given through coauthorship, acknowledgment, footnote statement, or other appropriate means, in accordance with such contributions. (See G.4.b. and G.4.c.)

e. Close Relatives. Counselors do not accept close relatives as students or supervisees.

f. Supervision Preparation. Counselors who offer clinical supervision services are adequately prepared in supervision methods and techniques. Counselors who are doctoral students serving as practicum or internship supervisors to master's level students are adequately prepared and supervised by the training program.

g. Responsibility for Services to Clients. Counselors who supervise the counseling services of others take reasonable measures to ensure that counseling services provided to clients are professional.

h. Endorsement. Counselors do not endorse students or supervisees for certification, licensure, employment, or completion of an academic or training program if they believe students or supervisees are not qualified for the endorsement. Counselors take reasonable steps to assist students or supervisees who are not qualified for endorsement to become qualified.

F.2. Counselor Education and Training Programs

a. Orientation. Prior to admission, counselors orient prospective students to the counselor education or training program's expectations, including but not limited to the following: (1) the type and level of skill acquisition required for successful completion of the training, (2) subject matter to be covered, (3) basis for evaluation, (4) training components that encourage self-growth or self-disclosure as part of the training process, (5) the type of supervision settings and requirements of the sites for required clinical field experiences, (6) student and supervisee evaluation and dismissal policies and procedures, and (7) up-to-date employment prospects for graduates.

b. Integration of Study and Practice. Counselors establish counselor education and training programs that integrate academic study and supervised practice.

c. Evaluation. Counselors clearly state to students and supervisees, in advance of training, the levels of competency expected, appraisal methods, and timing of evaluations for both didactic and experiential components. Counselors provide students and supervisees with periodic performance appraisal and evaluation feedback throughout the training program.

d. Teaching Ethics. Counselors make students and supervisees aware of the ethical responsibilities and standards of the profession and the students' and supervisees' ethical responsibilities to the profession. (See C.1. and F.3.e.)

e. Peer Relationships. When students or supervisees are assigned to lead counseling groups or provide clinical supervision for their peers, counselors take steps to ensure that students and supervisees placed in these roles do not have personal or adverse relationships with peers and that they understand they have the same ethical obligations as counselor educators, trainers, and supervisors. Counselors make every effort to ensure that the rights of peers are not compromised when students or supervisees are assigned to lead counseling groups or provide clinical supervision.

f. Varied Theoretical Positions. Counselors present varied theoretical positions so that students and supervisees may make comparisons and have opportunities to develop their own positions. Counselors provide information concerning the scientific bases of professional practice. (See C.6.a.)

g. Field Placements. Counselors develop clear policies within their training program regarding field placement and other clinical experiences. Counselors provide clearly stated roles and responsibilities for the student or supervisee, the site supervisor, and the program supervisor. They confirm that site supervisors are qualified to provide supervision and are informed of their professional and ethical responsibilities in this role.

h. Dual Relationships as Supervisors. Counselors avoid dual relationships such as performing the role of site supervisor and training program supervisor in the student's or supervisee's training program. Counselors do not accept any form of professional services, fees, commissions, reimbursement, or remuneration from a site for student or supervisee placement.

(continued)

RESOURCE V CONTINUED

i. Diversity in Programs. Counselors are responsive to their institution's and program's recruitment and retention needs for training program administrators, faculty, and students with diverse backgrounds and special needs. (See A.2.a.)

F.3. Students and Supervisees

a. Limitations. Counselors, through ongoing evaluation and appraisal, are aware of the academic and personal limitations of students and supervisees that might impede performance. Counselors assist students and supervisees in securing remedial assistance when needed, and dismiss from the training program supervisees who are unable to provide competent service due to academic or personal limitations. Counselors seek professional consultation and document their decision to dismiss or refer students or supervisees for assistance. Counselors ensure that students and supervisees have recourse to address decisions made to require them to seek assistance or to dismiss them.

b. Self-Growth Experiences. Counselors use professional judgment when designing training experiences conducted by the counselors themselves that require student and supervisee self-growth or self-disclosure. Safeguards are provided so that students and supervisees are aware of the ramifications their self-disclosure may have on counselors whose primary role as teacher, trainer, or supervisor requires acting on ethical obligations to the profession. Evaluative components of experiential training experiences explicitly delineate predetermined academic standards that are separate and do not depend on the student's level of self-disclosure. (See A.6.)

c. Counseling for Students and Supervisees. If students or supervisees request counseling, supervisors or counselor educators provide them with acceptable referrals. Supervisors or counselor educators do not serve as counselor to students or supervisees over whom they hold administrative, teaching, or evaluative roles unless this is a brief role associated with a training experience. (See A.6.b.)

d. Clients of Students and Supervisees. Counselors make every effort to ensure that the clients at field placements are aware of the services rendered and the qualifications of the students and supervisees rendering those services. Clients receive professional disclosure information and are informed of the limits of confidentiality. Client permission is obtained in order for the students and supervisees to use any information concerning the counseling relationship in the training process. (See B.1.e.)

e. Standards for Students and Supervisees. Students and supervisees preparing to become counselors adhere to the Code of Ethics and the Standards of Practice. Students and supervisees have the same obligations to clients as those required of counselors. (See H.1.)

Section G: Research and Publication

G.1. Research Responsibilities

a. Use of Human Subjects. Counselors plan, design, conduct, and report research in a manner consistent with pertinent ethical principles, federal and state laws, host institutional regulations, and scientific standards governing research with human subjects. Counselors design and conduct research that reflects cultural sensitivity appropriateness.

b. Deviation From Standard Practices. Counselors seek consultation and observe stringent safeguards to protect the rights of research participants when a research problem suggests a deviation from standard acceptable practices. (See B.6.)

c. Precautions to Avoid Injury. Counselors who conduct research with human subjects are responsible for the subjects' welfare throughout the experiment and take reasonable precautions to avoid causing injurious psychological, physical, or social effects to their subjects.

d. Principal Researcher Responsibility. The ultimate responsibility for ethical research practice lies with the principal researcher. All others involved in the research activities share ethical obligations and full responsibility for their own actions.

e. Minimal Interference. Counselors take reasonable precautions to avoid causing disruptions in subjects' lives due to participation in research.

f. Diversity. Counselors are sensitive to diversity and research issues with special populations. They seek consultation when appropriate. (See A.2.a. and B.6.)

G.2. Informed Consent

a. Topics Disclosed. In obtaining informed consent for research, counselors use language that is understandable to research participants and that (1) accurately explains the purpose and procedures to be followed; (2) identifies any procedures that are experimental or relatively untried; (3) describes the attendant discomforts and risks; (4) describes the benefits or changes in individuals or organizations that might be reasonably expected; (5) discloses appropriate alternative procedures that would be advantageous for subjects; (6) offers to answer any inquiries concerning the procedures; (7) describes any limitations on confidentiality;

(continued)

RESOURCE V CONTINUED

and (8) instructs that subjects are free to withdraw their consent and to discontinue participation in the project at any time. (See B.1.f.)

b. Deception. Counselors do not conduct research involving deception unless alternative procedures are not feasible and the prospective value of the research justifies the deception. When the methodological requirements of a study necessitate concealment or deception, the investigator is required to explain clearly the reasons for this action as soon as possible.

c. Voluntary Participation. Participation in research is typically voluntary and without any penalty for refusal to participate. Involuntary participation is appropriate only when it can be demonstrated that participation will have no harmful effects on subjects and is essential to the investigation.

d. Confidentiality of Information. Information obtained about research participants during the course of an investigation is confidential. When the possibility exists that others may obtain access to such information, ethical research practice requires that the possibility, together with the plans for protecting confidentiality, be explained to participants as a part of the procedure for obtaining informed consent. (See B.1.e.)

e. Persons Incapable of Giving Informed Consent. When a person is incapable of giving informed consent, counselors provide an appropriate explanation, obtain agreement for participation, and obtain appropriate consent from a legally authorized person.

f. Commitments to Participants. Counselors take reasonable measures to honor all commitments to research participants.

g. Explanations After Data Collection. After data are collected, counselors provide participants with full clarification of the nature of the study to remove any misconceptions. Where scientific or human values justify delaying or withholding information, counselors take reasonable measures to avoid causing harm.

h. Agreements to Cooperate. Counselors who agree to cooperate with another individual in research or publication incur an obligation to cooperate as promised in terms of punctuality of performance and with regard to the completeness and accuracy of the information required.

i. Informed Consent for Sponsors. In the pursuit of research, counselors give sponsors, institutions, and publication channels the same respect and opportunity for giving informed consent that they accord to individual research participants. Counselors are aware of their obligation to future research workers and ensure that host institutions are given feedback information and proper acknowledgment.

G.3. Reporting Results

a. Information Affecting Outcome. When reporting research results, counselors explicitly mention all variables and conditions known to the investigator that may have affected the outcome of a study or the interpretation of data.

b. Accurate Results. Counselors plan, conduct, and report research accurately and in a manner that minimizes the possibility that results will be misleading. They provide thorough discussions of the limitations of their data and alternative hypotheses. Counselors do not engage in fraudulent research, distort data, misrepresent data, or deliberately bias their results.

c. Obligation to Report Unfavorable Results. Counselors communicate to other counselors the results of any research judged to be of professional value. Results that reflect unfavorably on institutions, programs, services, prevailing opinions, or vested interests are not withheld.

d. Identity of Subjects. Counselors who supply data, aid in the research of another person, report research results, or make original data available take due care to disguise the identity of respective subjects in the absence of specific authorization from the subjects to do otherwise. (See B.1.g. and B.5.a.)

e. Replication Studies. Counselors are obligated to make available sufficient original research data to qualified professionals who may wish to replicate the study.

G.4. Publication

a. Recognition of Others. When conducting and reporting research, counselors are familiar with and give recognition to previous work on the topic, observe copyright laws, and give full credit to those to whom credit is due. (See F.1.d. and G.4.c.)

b. Contributors. Counselors give credit through joint authorship, acknowledgment, footnote statements, or other appropriate means to those who have contributed significantly to research or concept development in accordance with such contributions. The principal contributor is listed first and minor technical or professional contributions are acknowledged in notes or introductory statements.

c. Student Research. For an article that is substantially based on a student's dissertation or thesis, the student is listed as the principal author. (See F.1.d. and G.4.a.)

d. Duplicate Submission. Counselors submit manuscripts for consideration to only one journal at a time. Manuscripts that are published in whole or in substantial part in another journal or

(continued)

RESOURCE V CONTINUED

published work are not submitted for publication without acknowledgment and permission from the previous publication.

   e. Professional Review. Counselors who review material submitted
for publication, research, or other scholarly purposes respect the
confidentiality and proprietary rights of those who submitted it.

Section H: Resolving Ethical Issues

H.1. Knowledge of Standards
Counselors are familiar with the Code of Ethics and the Standards
of Practice and other applicable ethics codes from other professional organizations of which they are member, or from certification and licensure bodies. Lack of knowledge or misunderstanding
of an ethical responsibility is not a defense against a charge of unethical conduct. (See F.3.e.)

H.2. Suspected Violations

   a. Ethical Behavior Expected. Counselors expect professional associates to adhere to the Code of Ethics. When counselors possess
reasonable cause that raises doubts as to whether a counselor is
acting in an ethical manner, they take appropriate action. (See
H.2.d. and H.2.e.)

   b. Consultation. When uncertain as to whether a particular situation
or course of action may be in violation of the Code of Ethics,
counselors consult with other counselors who are knowledgeable
about ethics, with colleagues, or with appropriate authorities.

   c. Organization Conflicts. If the demands of an organization with
which counselors are affiliated pose a conflict with the Code of
Ethics, counselors specify the nature of such conflicts and express to their supervisors or other responsible officials their commitment to the Code of Ethics. When possible, counselors work
toward change within the organization to allow full adherence to
the Code of Ethics.

   d. Informal Resolution. When counselors have reasonable cause to
believe that another counselor is violating an ethical standard,
they attempt to first resolve the issue informally with the other
counselor if feasible, providing that such action does not violate
confidentiality rights that may be involved.

   e. Reporting Suspected Violations. When an informal resolution is
not appropriate or feasible, counselors, upon reasonable cause,
take action such as reporting the suspected ethical violation to
state or national ethics committees, unless this action conflicts
with confidentiality rights that cannot be resolved.

     f. Unwarranted Complaints. Counselors do not initiate, participate in, or encourage the filing of ethics complaints that are unwarranted or intend to harm a counselor rather than to protect clients or the public.

H.3. Cooperation With Ethics Committees
Counselors assist in the process of enforcing the Code of Ethics. Counselors cooperate with investigations, proceedings, and requirements of the ACA Ethics Committee or ethics committees of other duly constituted associations or boards having jurisdiction over those charged with a violation. Counselors are familiar with the ACA Policies and Procedures and use it as a reference in assisting the enforcement of the Code of Ethics.

ACA Standards of Practice

All members of the American Counseling Association (ACA) are required to adhere to the Standards of Practice and the Code of Ethics. The Standards of Practice represent minimal behavioral statements of the Code of Ethics. Members should refer to the applicable section of the Code of Ethics for further interpretation and amplification of the applicable Standard of Practice.

Section A: The Counseling Relationship
Section B: Confidentiality
Section C: Professional Responsibility
Section D: Relationship With Other Professionals
Section E: Evaluation, Assessment and Interpretation
Section F: Teaching, Training, and Supervision
Section G: Research and Publication
Section H: Resolving Ethical Issues

Section A: The Counseling Relationship

STANDARD OF PRACTICE ONE (SP-1): Nondiscrimination. Counselors respect diversity and must not discriminate against clients because of age, color, culture, disability, ethnic group, gender, race, religion, sexual orientation, marital status, or socioeconomic status. (See A.2.a.)

STANDARD OF PRACTICE TWO (SP-2): Disclosure to Clients. Counselors must adequately inform clients, preferably in writing, regarding the counseling process and counseling relationship at or before the time it begins and throughout the relationship. (See A.3.a.)

STANDARD OF PRACTICE THREE (SP-3): Dual Relationships. Counselors must make every effort to avoid dual relationships with clients that could impair their professional judgment or increase the risk of harm to clients. When a dual relationship cannot be avoided, counselors must take appropriate steps to ensure that judgment is not impaired and that no exploitation occurs. (See A.6.a. and A.6.b.)

(continued)

RESOURCE V CONTINUED

STANDARD OF PRACTICE FOUR (SP-4):   Sexual Intimacies With Clients. Counselors must not engage in any type of sexual intimacies with current clients and must not engage in sexual intimacies with former clients within a minimum of 2 years after terminating the counseling relationship. Counselors who engage in such relationship after 2 years following termination have the responsibility to examine and document thoroughly that such relations did not have an exploitative nature.

STANDARD OF PRACTICE FIVE (SP-5):   Protecting Clients During Group Work. Counselors must take steps to protect clients from physical or psychological trauma resulting from interactions during group work. (See A.9.b.)

STANDARD OF PRACTICE SIX (SP-6):   Advance Understanding of Fees. Counselors must explain to clients, prior to their entering the counseling relationship, financial arrangements related to professional services. (See A.10. a.-d. and A.11.c.)

STANDARD OF PRACTICE SEVEN (SP-7):   Termination. Counselors must assist in making appropriate arrangements for the continuation of treatment of clients, when necessary, following termination of counseling relationships. (See A.11.a.)

STANDARD OF PRACTICE EIGHT (SP-8):   Inability to Assist Clients. Counselors must avoid entering or immediately terminate a counseling relationship if it is determined that they are unable to be of professional assistance to a client. The counselor may assist in making an appropriate referral for the client. (See A.11.b.)

Section B: Confidentiality

STANDARD OF PRACTICE NINE (SP-9):   Confidentiality Requirement. Counselors must keep information related to counseling services confidential unless disclosure is in the best interest of clients, is required for the welfare of others, or is required by law. When disclosure is required, only information that is essential is revealed and the client is informed of such disclosure. (See B.1. a. and f.)

STANDARD OF PRACTICE TEN (SP-10):   Confidentiality Requirements for Subordinates. Counselors must take measures to ensure that privacy and confidentiality of clients are maintained by subordinates. (See B.1.h.)

STANDARD OF PRACTICE ELEVEN (SP-11):   Confidentiality in Group Work. Counselors must clearly communicate to group members that confidentiality cannot be guaranteed in group work. (See B.2.a.)

STANDARD OF PRACTICE TWELVE (SP-12):   Confidentiality in Family Counseling. Counselors must not disclose information about one family member in counseling to another family member without prior consent. (See B.2.b.)

STANDARD OF PRACTICE THIRTEEN (SP-13): Confidentiality of Records. Counselors must maintain appropriate confidentiality in creating, storing, accessing, transferring, and disposing of counseling records. (See B.4.b.)

STANDARD OF PRACTICE FOURTEEN (SP-14): Permission to Record or Observe. Counselors must obtain prior consent from clients in order to record electronically or observe sessions. (See B.4.c.)

STANDARD OF PRACTICE FIFTEEN (SP-15): Disclosure or Transfer of Records. Counselors must obtain client consent to disclose or transfer records to third parties, unless exceptions listed in SP-9 exist. (See B.4.e.)

STANDARD OF PRACTICE SIXTEEN (SP-16): Data Disguise Required. Counselors must disguise the identity of the client when using data for training, research, or publication. (See B.5.a.)

Section C: Professional Responsibility

STANDARD OF PRACTICE SEVENTEEN (SP-17): Boundaries of Competence. Counselors must practice only within the boundaries of their competence. (See C.2.a.)

STANDARD OF PRACTICE EIGHTEEN (SP-18): Continuing Education. Counselors must engage in continuing education to maintain their professional competence. (See C.2.f.)

STANDARD OF PRACTICE NINETEEN (SP-19): Impairment of Professionals. Counselors must refrain from offering professional services when their personal problems or conflicts may cause harm to a client or others. (See C.2.g.)

STANDARD OF PRACTICE TWENTY (SP-20): Accurate Advertising. Counselors must accurately represent their credentials and services when advertising. (See C.3.a.)

STANDARD OF PRACTICE TWENTY-ONE (SP-21): Recruiting Through Employment. Counselors must not use their place of employment or institutional affiliation to recruit clients for their private practices. (See C.3.d.)

STANDARD OF PRACTICE TWENTY-TWO (SP-22): Credentials Claimed. Counselors must claim or imply only professional credentials possessed and must correct any known misrepresentations of their credentials by others. (See C.4.a.)

STANDARD OF PRACTICE TWENTY-THREE (SP-23): Sexual Harassment. Counselors must not engage in sexual harassment. (See C.5.b.)

STANDARD OF PRACTICE TWENTY-FOUR (SP-24): Unjustified Gains. Counselors must not use their professional positions to seek or receive unjustified personal gains, sexual favors, unfair advantage, or unearned goods or services. (See C.5.e.)

STANDARD OF PRACTICE TWENTY-FIVE (SP-25): Clients Served by Others. With the consent of the client, counselors must inform other mental

(continued)

RESOURCE V CONTINUED

health professionals serving the same client that a counseling relationship between the counselor and client exists. (See C.6.c.)

STANDARD OF PRACTICE TWENTY-SIX (SP-26): Negative Employment Conditions. Counselors must alert their employers to institutional policy or conditions that may be potentially disruptive or damaging to the counselor's professional responsibilities, or that may limit their effectiveness or deny clients' rights. (See D.1.c.)

STANDARD OF PRACTICE TWENTY-SEVEN (SP-27): Personnel Selection and Assignment. Counselors must select competent staff and must assign responsibilities compatible with staff skills and experiences. (See D.1.h.)

STANDARD OF PRACTICE TWENTY-EIGHT (SP-28): Exploitative Relationships With Subordinates. Counselors must not engage in exploitative relationships with individuals over whom they have supervisory, evaluative, or instructional control or authority. (See D.1.k.)

Section D: Relationship With Other Professionals

STANDARD OF PRACTICE TWENTY-NINE (SP-29): Accepting Fees From Agency Clients. Counselors must not accept fees or other remuneration for consultation with persons entitled to such services through the counselor's employing agency or institution. (See D.3.a.)

STANDARD OF PRACTICE THIRTY (SP-30): Referral Fees. Counselors must not accept referral fees. (See D.3.b.)

Section E: Evaluation, Assesment and Interpretation

STANDARD OF PRACTICE THIRTY-ONE (SP-31): Limits of Competence. Counselors must perform only testing and assessment services for which they are competent. Counselors must not allow the use of psychological assessment techniques by unqualified persons under their supervision. (See E.2.a.)

STANDARD OF PRACTICE THIRTY-TWO (SP-32): Appropriate Use of Assessment Instruments. Counselors must use assessment instruments in the manner for which they were intended. (See E.2.b.)

STANDARD OF PRACTICE THIRTY-THREE (SP-33): Assessment Explanations to Clients. Counselors must provide explanations to clients prior to assessment about the nature and purposes of assessment and the specific uses of results. (See E.3.a.)

STANDARD OF PRACTICE THIRTY-FOUR (SP-34): Recipients of Test Results. Counselors must ensure that accurate and appropriate interpretations accompany any release of testing and assessment information. (See E.3.b.)

STANDARD OF PRACTICE THIRTY-FIVE (SP-35): Obsolete Tests and Outdated Test Results. Counselors must not base their assessment or intervention decisions or recommendations on data or test results that are obsolete or outdated for the current purpose. (See E.11.)

Section F: Teaching, Training, and Supervision

STANDARD OF PRACTICE THIRTY-SIX (SP-36):   Sexual Relationships With Students or Supervisees. Counselors must not engage in sexual relationships with their students and supervisees. (See F.1.c.)

STANDARD OF PRACTICE THIRTY-SEVEN (SP-37):   Credit for Contributions to Research. Counselors must give credit to students or supervisees for their contributions to research and scholarly projects. (See F.1.d.)

STANDARD OF PRACTICE THIRTY-EIGHT (SP-38):   Supervision Preparation. Counselors who offer clinical supervision services must be trained and prepared in supervision methods and techniques. (See F.1.f.)

STANDARD OF PRACTICE THIRTY-NINE (SP-39):   Evaluation Information. Counselors must clearly state to students and supervisees in advance of training the levels of competency expected, appraisal methods, and timing of evaluations. Counselors must provide students and supervisees with periodic performance appraisal and evaluation feedback throughout the training program. (See F.2.c.)

STANDARD OF PRACTICE FORTY (SP-40):   Peer Relationships in Training. Counselors must make every effort to ensure that the rights of peers are not violated when students and supervisees are assigned to lead counseling groups or provide clinical supervision. (See F.2.e.)

STANDARD OF PRACTICE FORTY-ONE (SP-41):   Limitations of Students and Supervisees. Counselors must assist students and supervisees in securing remedial assistance, when needed, and must dismiss from the training program students and supervisees who are unable to provide competent service due to academic or personal limitations. (See F.3.a.)

STANDARD OF PRACTICE FORTY-TWO (SP-42):   Self-Growth Experiences. Counselors who conduct experiences for students or supervisees that include self-growth or self-disclosure must inform participants of counselors' ethical obligations to the profession and must not grade participants based on their nonacademic performance. (See F.3.b.)

STANDARD OF PRACTICE FORTY-THREE (SP-43):   Standards for Students and Supervisees. Students and supervisees preparing to become counselors must adhere to the Code of Ethics and the Standards of Practice of counselors. (See F.3.e.)

Section G: Research and Publication

STANDARD OF PRACTICE FORTY-FOUR (SP-44):   Precautions to Avoid Injury in Research. Counselors must avoid causing physical, social, or psychological harm or injury to subjects in research. (See G.1.c.)

(continued)

RESOURCE V CONTINUED

STANDARD OF PRACTICE FORTY-FIVE (SP-45): Confidentiality of research information. counselors must keep confidential information obtained about research participants. (See G.2.d.)

STANDARD OF PRACTICE FORTY-SIX (SP-46): Information Affecting Research Outcome. Counselors must report all variables and conditions known to the investigator that may have affected research data or outcomes. (See G.3.a.)

STANDARD OF PRACTICE FORTY-SEVEN (SP-47): Accurate Research Results. Counselors must not distort or misrepresent research data, nor fabricate or intentionally bias research results. (See G.3.b.)

STANDARD OF PRACTICE FORTY-EIGHT (SP-48): Publication Contributors. Counselors must give appropriate credit to those who have contributed to research. (See G.4.a. and G.4.b.)

Section H: Resolving Ethical Issues

STANDARD OF PRACTICE FORTY-NINE (SP-49): Ethical Behavior Expected. Counselors must take appropriate action when they possess reasonable cause that raises doubts as to whether counselors or other mental health professionals are acting in an ethical manner. (See H.2.a.)

STANDARD OF PRACTICE FIFTY (SP-50): Unwarranted Complaints. Counselors must not initiate, participate in, or encourage the filing of ethics complaints that are unwarranted or intended to harm a mental health professional rather than to protect clients or the public. (See H.2.f.)

STANDARD OF PRACTICE FIFTY-ONE (SP-51): Cooperation With Ethics Committees. Counselors must cooperate with investigations, proceedings, and requirements of the ACA Ethics Committee or ethics committees of other duly constituted associations or boards having jurisdiction over those charged with a violation. (See H.3.)

References

The following documents are available to counselors as resources to guide them in their practices. These resources are not a part of the Code of Ethics and the Standards of Practice.

American Association for Counseling and Development/Association for Measurement and Evaluation in Counseling and Development. (1989). The responsibilities of users of standardized tests (rev.). Washington, DC:

American Counseling Association. (1995) (Note: This is ACA's previous edition of its ethics code). Ethical standards. Alexandria, VA:

COUNSELING RESEARCH OUTCOMES: DISCOVERING WHAT WORKS

☞ *Using evidence-based research will ensure that you are conducting quality counseling. As counselors our goal is to change some type of (problematic) behavior, thought, or feeling. Measuring behavioral change is one accountable way of assessing whether change has occurred (Vicky White, 2002).*

OVERVIEW

GOALS

KEY CONCEPTS: PRACTICING EVIDENCE-BASED COUNSELING

A BRIEF HISTORY OF COUNSELING EFFECTIVENESS AND CHANGE
PRACTICAL REFLECTION 1: BEGINNING TO PRACTICE OUTCOME RESEARCH

TYPES OF OUTCOME RESEARCH
DESCRIPTIVE RESEARCH
QUANTITATIVE DESIGNS
PROGRAM, CLIENT, COUNSELOR, AND SUPERVISION EVALUATIONS
META-ANALYSIS

QUALITATIVE DESIGNS
PRACTICAL REFLECTION 2: SELECTING THE MOST EFFICIENT RESEARCH TYPE FOR YOU

RESEARCH PRACTITIONER MODELS
SCIENTIST/PRACTITIONER MODEL
PRACTICAL REFLECTION 3: CLARIFYING YOUR STRENGTHS AND LIABILITIES
TEACHER/SCHOLAR MODEL
PRACTICAL REFLECTION 4: CHOOSING YOUR BEST FIT SCHOLARLY FUNCTION

SUMMARY AND PERSONAL INTEGRATION
PRACTICAL REFLECTION 5: INTEGRATION

REFERENCES
RESOURCE W

OVERVIEW

Much of the research on counseling effectiveness has been theoretically based and historical. This chapter discusses action research that is outcome based and summarizes the need for quality evaluation procedures for the counseling and supervision process. You will be asked to integrate approaches and evaluations that will make your counseling more accountable and effective.

GOALS

1. Understand the need for counseling outcome research or evidence-based counseling practices.
2. Examine differing methods for conducting your own outcome research.
3. Evaluate consistently your counseling effectiveness and that of your supervisors and clients.
4. Commit to consistent use of personal, clinical, and client evaluations.

KEY CONCEPTS: PRACTICING EVIDENCE-BASED COUNSELING

It is our ethical and professional responsibility to understand what makes counseling effective. These days of managed care have made us more aware of our efficacy and called for accountability of our services (Hayes, Barlow, & Nelson-Gray, 1999; Whiston, 1996). It is also important that you investigate not only the efficacy of counseling but also the validity of psychotherapy (Mace & Moorey, 2001). You must be realistic in what outcome research has to offer (Lambert, 2003).

Clients must be given the highest standards of care by receiving the best practices; as a new helping professional, you must be able to determine if, how, and when your clients change (Snyder & Ingrams, 2000). One day a discussion in our counseling internship class evolved concerning client termination. I was emphasizing the importance of creating a therapeutic atmosphere that encourages setting of client counseling goals, evaluation of those goals, and appropriate termination, all at the very beginning of the counseling relationship. A brave intern stammered, "I never seem to get to the termination phase, and exactly how do you know when a client has completed counseling?" The class was very quiet, and soon other students nodded their heads, as if to thank the student for asking a question that was on all their minds! From that conversation came the foundation for understanding the essentials of client change, action research, and program evaluation.

A Brief History of Counseling Effectiveness and Change

For many years, researchers have been discussing whether counseling interventions have been effective. Do you remember hearing about the Eysenck debates in the 1960s? Eysenck (1966) stated that counseling was not effective. This caused much controversy in the helping professions and sparked the need for better research.

In *The Benefits of Psychotherapy*, Smith, Glass, and Miller (1980) used a meta-analysis to evaluate the effectiveness of counseling interventions. They found that counseling interventions were more effective in 80 percent of subjects when compared to a control group. In this study, theoretical orientation did not seem to make a difference, but empathy in the counseling relationship did.

Lambert and Cattani-Thompson (1996) researched counseling effectiveness and change. They found that client variables accounted for 64 percent of the change. Client variables were described as severity of disturbances, motivation, capacity to relate, ego strength, psychological mindedness, and ability to clearly identify problems. Relationship factors, such as therapeutic relationships and past and present personal relationships, accounted for approximately 30 percent of change. Specific interventions chosen to address specific problems and concerns accounted for 6 percent of change.

Counseling Outcome Research: Investigations of counseling problems that lead to causal, relational, and/or attitudinal answers about counseling effectiveness.

Outcome-based counseling research is becoming more common, expected, and accessible (Mace, Moorey & Roberts, 2001). There appear to be three counseling outcome research questions that need to be consistently addressed (Elliott, 2002). First, you must ask yourself, "Has my client actually changed?" (Elliott, 2002; Strupp, Horowitz, & Lambert, 1997). If the answer is yes, a second outcome research question needs to be addressed: Was it the actual counseling that was responsible for my client's change? (Elliott, 2002; Haaga & Stiles, 2000). If the answer to the first question is no, then you must ask, "Why was there no change?" Then a final question needs to be analyzed: What direct or indirect factors or evidence are responsible for the change? (Eliott, 2002; Greenburg, 1986). For example changes may be attributed to statistical and research biases, counseling relationship biases, client expectations, client self-correction, events that occurred outside of counseling, and medication benefits. See

> ## Practical Reflection 1: Beginning to Practice Outcome Research
>
> Describe what you are currently doing to integrate outcome research into your counseling interventions. What research questions are you asking about your counseling effectiveness?
>
> _____
> _____
> _____
> _____

Evidence-Based Counseling Practice: Best practice techniques and measures that come from counseling outcome research.

Resource W for more detail of the eight indirect evidence methods evaluating the possible nontherapy explanations.

Whether these questions are researched qualitatively, quantitatively, or both may not be realistic for your counseling agency or practice. However, you owe it to yourself and your clients to at least ask these questions in supervision by taking the skeptic's position that counseling was not responsible or the affirmative side that counseling did make a difference (Eliott, 2002). That would be a beginning for you toward evidence-based counseling practice.

TYPES OF OUTCOME RESEARCH

There are many different types of available outcome research for you to choose and utilize (Heppner, Kivlighan, & Wampold, 1999). Your task is to find the kinds that are best suited for your counseling practice and client populations. In a survey designed by Sexton (1996), the five most popular types of research presented are descriptive fields, quantitative/experimental designs, program evaluations, meta-analysis, and qualitative analysis. Let's take a brief look at those five selected methods of conducting outcome research. These descriptions will be skeletal in nature and very selective. There are numerous additional types of research, so be sure to go back to your basic research and statistics coursework for a more thorough review.

Descriptive Research

Research studies that use descriptive fields generally offer readers information concerning measures of central tendencies. Statistics on the mean, mode, median, standard deviations, and more are usually presented. The main function of descriptive studies is to describe what the population being studied actually are like.

In your counseling practice, you might use descriptive fields to count the number of times your client attended his or her scheduled interviews. Perhaps you wanted to target a certain symptomatic behavior and count the number of times your client reported a decrease or increase in that targeted behavior.

Using descriptive fields is an endless method of collecting essential information and demographics. If nothing else, you might use descriptive statistics to list the type of clients you are seeing, the ratio of males to females, the average age of your clientele, or even the types of problems you are seeing the most. You could also use descriptive research to tell if you are seeing women for 10 sessions, but you only see men for 3. You could track whether your culturally different clients drop out sooner than others. By now you can tell that this method of data collection is essential to your counseling practice.

Quantitative Designs

Quantitative Research:
Research designed to find the truth through the scientific method of deduction.

Through the scientific method, quantitative research designs surmise that possible answers to research hypotheses or questions can be discovered. There are two types of quantitative research: experimental and nonexperimental. *Experimental research* searches for cause and effect by manipulating the treatment variables. *Nonexperimental research* often looks at relationships between variables (Neukrug, 1999).

Single-Case Designs:
A method of quantitative research where only one subject is studied.

One example of a quantitative, experimental method relevant to counseling is the single subject/case design. Single-case and $N = 1$ designs are natural units for most clinical practices because they are practical and applicable to clients. Because you cannot generalize from group research to individual clients, the use of single-case designs has rationality and clinical utility (Elliott, 2002; Lundervold & Belwood, 2000).

You could take almost any one of your clients and develop a single-case study. If your client came to you with the presenting problem of anxiety and procrastination in completing work projects, you would follow three basic steps. First a baseline would need to be measured using a valid and reliable instrument for anxiety and procrastination, labeled (A).

Then a treatment for anxiety and procrastination would be offered over the next few weeks, labeled (B). Measurements during the treatment would be taken. Finally after the treatment is over, the same measurements (A) would be taken to see if the treatment had, in fact, reduced the anxiety and procrastination over completing work projects. If you wanted to extend your study you may prefer to use the ABAB model. This is one of many examples of a quantitative, experimental method using a single-case design. Elliott's (2002) essential research questions can be applied to this ABA or ABAB single-case study as well.

Program, Client, Counselor, and Supervision Evaluations

Evaluations are crucial to the effectiveness of your counseling practice and your counseling skills. Evaluations are another method of determining whether or not a program or intervention has been an effective counseling strategy for change.

There are several ways to accomplish program evaluations. Once you have determined the specific concern, you could select a pre- and posttest method using a valid and reliable instrument such as the Beck Depression Inventory that measures the diagnosed problem of depression in your client.

It is also essential to evaluate your individual and group clients. Patterson and Basham (2002) conducted a study creating graphs for weekly group evaluations to track individual and group results with promising results. Other researchers have found group evaluations informative with women's issues and career concerns (Sullivan & Mahalik, 2000; Marlotta & Asner, 1999).

As counselors we do not perform enough of this type of evaluation. This evaluation is easy to accomplish, though, as you can and should be evaluating at the end of every counseling session! I also assess the individual counseling goals at the end of every three sessions. Both methods assist you and the client in determining the efficacy of the counseling sessions. These evaluations do not determine whether it was the actual counseling that caused change, but it will assist you in gathering the client's perceptions about change that occurred during the counseling period.

Be sure to allow time for you and your counseling supervisor to assess your progress. One effective way to conduct evaluations is to examine your own use of skills. In previous chapters, you used the Counseling Interview Rating Form (CIRF) to rate and classify your counseling skills. This is one method of using process research to analyze your skills. You may want to periodically review your interviewing style and submit it to colleagues and supervisors at least annually. Both of these evaluations will keep you fresh and challenged!

Ask your supervisor if she or he will be willing to receive feedback from you on a regular basis. Ask your supervisors and instructors for examples to guide you. Some supervisors may have little experience and education in supervision and may be reluctant and naïve about the supervision process (Magnuson, Wilcoxen, & Norem, 2000). You may want and need to develop your own evaluations that will better reflect personal needs relevant to your counseling practice.

Meta-Analysis

The positive attribute of meta-analysis is clear: it allows you to synthesize research data from many projects over time in an aggregate manner. Recently the methods of meta analysis have become more discriminating and useful (Mace & Moorey, 2001). In your counseling work you could look to see whether the effect size of a certain program on substance abuse has proven effective over its 10-year history.

Qualitative Designs

Qualitative Research: Research discoveries that have a naturalistic-phenomenological approach (Schumacher & McMillan, 1993).

Qualitative research presumes that there are many different ways to experience and interpret the world. The scientific method may not be able to answer all the different realities that a person may perceive, such as abstractions and meanings. The qualitative researcher becomes a careful observer of a phenomenon and begins to describe and interpret its attitudinal and sociological contexts (Kopala & Suzuki, 1999; Neukrug, 1999).

Behavioral Observations: A type of qualitative research where observations are noted, reviewed and interpreted.

One type of qualitative study is the Behavorial Observation Plan. This method can be very helpful to you in determining client change. There are many unique types of behavioral observations, but the eight steps to this plan can be used for a variety of purposes (Hayes, Barlow, & Nelson-Gray, 1999).

1. Conduct a preliminary assessment.
2. Determine the target behaviors.
3. Decide what and how many behaviors to record.
4. Decide who will observe and record the behaviors: client, counselor.
5. Decide when and where to record.
6. Train the observer.
7. Look at the concern in a systematic fashion.
8. Begin collecting baseline behavior.

For example, in the Case of Darryl, Step 1 was conducted by investigating his past and current behaviors. As the case was conceptualized and many problems surfaced, the goal of working on two coping skills was determined. Step 2 required that a target behavior be selected. For Darryl, because he had kept his secrets for a very long time, sharing even every day thoughts and feelings was a challenge. The targeted behaviors for Darryl

Practical Reflection 2: Selecting the Most Efficient Research Type for You

---

Of the outcome research types mentioned, which method could you see yourself actually implementing in your counseling work? For example, could you see yourself using evaluations, the CIRF, single-case designs, or behavioral observation plans?

_____

_____

_____

_____

---

were to share at least two thoughts and feeling with his wife, Sophia, and his son, Michael. Darryl was asked to spend at least 15 minutes per day playing with Michael and sharing thoughts with Sophia. In Steps 3, 4, 5, and 6, Darryl recorded in a daily journal how he shared with his family.

Steps 7 and 8 began at the next counseling session. Information collected acts as a beginning phase determining Darryl's baseline behaviors and their outcomes. This same method could be used to track Darryl's nightmares and depressive symptoms.

RESEARCH PRACTITIONER MODELS

Now that you have had a review of some of the available types of outcome research, two theoretical models may help solidify your opinions and guide you into future research of your own. Here are two major models that can be used to assist the helping professions in becoming researchers as well as counselors. The first is the scientist/practitioner model and the second is the teacher/scholar paradigm.

Scientist/Practitioner Model

Scientist/Practitioner Model: A model where clinicians use outcome-based research and integrate into the world of counseling practice.

In this model, you as the helping professional must believe there are certain truths that will assist your client in changing thoughts and behaviors. You must also believe that you can discover additional truths about client change through research. In addition, as a counselor, you must have confidence in your skills to actually implement those truths into your therapy interventions.

Practical Reflection 3: Clarifying Your Strengths and Liabilities

What would be your biggest challenge in implementing the scientist/ practitioner model? How would this effect your counseling?

_____

_____

_____

_____

To use research in practice three things need to occur (Sexton & Whiston, 1996). Practitioners must be aware of what research is available. This statement reinforces how important it is that you join and maintain your professional affiliations. As you know, most of these associations provide you with newspapers and journals that keep abreast of the latest research, observations, and trends. Again your thoughts turn to time constraints. Just remember that you and your clients will benefit if you keep current in your specific discipline. The second skill is the ability to determine what the research you are reading actually means or what the implications are. You do not have to be an expert statistician, but you do need to know the basics related to quality research, whether the research is quantitative or qualitative. Last, you must make a commitment to yourself that you will consistently integrate your findings into your actual practice. If your current skills did not allow you to do so, be sure to get the skill training you may need to update your counseling interventions.

Teacher/Scholar Model

Teacher/Scholar Model: Boyer's (1990) model of diverse scholarly functions including discovery, integration, application, and teaching.

Many years ago I read the compelling work of Ernest Boyer (1990) entitled _Scholarship Reconsidered: Priorities of the Professoriate._ His ideas about the expanded functions of scholarship helped to crystallize the idea that counselors too can and must use scholarship to advance the profession of counseling. Boyer stated that scholarship had four unique but overlapping functions: the scholarship of discovery, the scholarship of integration, the scholarship of application, and the scholarship of teaching.

The _scholarship of discovery_ is the traditional meaning of research and asks the question, "What is yet to be known, what is yet to be found?"

Practical Reflection 4: Choosing Your Best Fit Scholarly Function

---

Which of Boyer's scholarly functions would best fit you and be compatible with your life as a new counseling practitioner? Choose one of the four and offer an example: scholarship of discovery, integration, application, or teaching.

_____

_____

_____

_____

(Boyer, 1990, p. 19). It adds to the knowledge base of the intellectual world. The *scholarship of integration* asks the question, "What do already existing findings means? Integration tends to be collaborative in nature and seeks to expand what past research has discovered. The *scholarship of application* moves even further and asks the question, "How can knowledge be applied to consequential problems?" (p. 21). Finally, the *scholarship of teaching* urges professors to ask the question, "How can we transmit knowledge creatively and in a challenging fashion?"

I have molded my university teaching career around these four separate functions, and I believe it has assisted me in becoming a well-rounded, dynamic, and versatile professor. These same scholarly functions can be used easily for you as a practicing counselor. Sometimes it seems that, as a practicing counselor, there is no time for research and scholarly production. We have to complete so many direct services hours to clients and the paperwork can be overwhelming! Using Boyer's expanded use of scholarship, you have many more options available to be a scholar as well as a counselor.

SUMMARY AND PERSONAL INTEGRATION

In this chapter, you were introduced to models and measures that could assist you in integrating outcome research into your counseling practice:

- The beginning step toward research awareness is to develop a commitment to evidence-based counseling practices or at least an orientation toward using it in your counseling practice.

Practical Reflection 5: Integration

Which of the constructs presented in this chapter will assist you in integrating research outcomes into your counseling practice?

_____

_____

_____

_____

- Knowing strengths and limitations of the research methods and studies chosen is essential.
- Being realistic in your expectations about what outcome research has to offer was recommended.
- Locating studies most similar to your particular counseling concern was recommended.
- The benefits of the scientist/practitioner and teacher/scholar models to your counseling practice were presented.
- Continue supervision whether it be individual or group counseling.

REFERENCES

Boyer, E. L. (1990). *Scholarship Reconsidered: Priorities of the Professoriate. Carnegie Foundation for the Advancement of Teaching*. San Francisco, CA: Jossey-Bass.

Elliott, R. (2002). Hermeneutic single-case efficacy design. *Psychotherapy Research, 12*, 1–21.

Elliott, R. (2002, May). Evaluating the effectiveness of therapy in your own practice: Hermeneutic single-case efficacy design. Paper presented at the British Association of Counselling and Psychotherapy Research Conference, London, England.

Eysenck, H. (1966). *The Effects of Psychotherapy*. New York: International Science Press.

Greenburg, L. S. (1986). Change process research. *Journal of Consulting and Clinical Psychology, 54*, 4–9.

Haaga, D. A., & Stiles, W. B. (2000). Randomized clinical trials in psychotherapy research: Methodology, design, and evaluation. In C. R. Snyder & R. E. Ingram. (Eds.). *Handbook of Psychological Change* (pp. 14–39). New York: John Wiley & Sons.

Hayes, S. C., Barlow, D. H., & Nelson-Gray, R. O. (Eds). (1999). *The Scientist-Practitioner: Research and Accountability in the Age of Managed Care* (2nd ed.). Boston: Allyn & Bacon.

Heppner, P. P., Kivlighan, D. M., & Wampold, B. E. (Eds.) (1999). *Research design in Counseling*. New York: Brooks/Cole.

Kopala, L. A. & Suzuki, M. (1999). Using qualitative methods in psychology. Thousand Oak, CA: Sage Publications.

Lambert, M. J. (2003). (5th ed). Bergin and Garfield's *Handbook of Psychotherapy and Behavior Change*. NY, NY: John Wiley & Sons, Inc.

Lambert, M. J., & Cattani-Thompson, K. (1996). Current findings regarding the effectiveness of counseling: Implications for practice. *Journal of Counseling and Development, 74*, 601–8.

Lundervold, D. A., & Belwood, M. F. (2000). The best kept secret in counseling: Single-case (*N* = 1) experimental designs. *Journal of Counseling and Development, 78*, 92–102.

Mace, C., & Moorey, S. (2001). Evidence in psychotherapy: A delicate balance. In C. Mace, S. Moorey, & B. Roberts. (Eds.). *Evidence in the Psychological Therapies* (pp. 1–11). East Sussex, Britain: Brunner-Routledge.

Mace, C., Moorey, S., & Roberts, B. (Eds.). (2001). *Evidence in the Psychological Therapies*. East Sussex, Britain: Brunner-Routledge.

Magnuson, S., Wilcoxen, A. S., & Norem, K. (2000). A profile of lousy supervision: Experienced counselors' perspectives. *Counselor Education and Supervision, 39*, 189–202.

Marotta, S. A., & Asner, K. K. (1999). Group psychotherapy for women with a history of incest: The research base. *Journal of Counseling and Development, 77*, 315–23.

Neukrug, E. (1999). *The World of the Counselor*. Pacific Grove, CA: Brooks/Cole.

Patterson, D., & Basham, R. (2002). A data visualization procedure for the evaluation of group treatment outcomes across units of analysis. *Small Group Research, 33*, 209–32.

Sexton, T. L. (1996). The relevance of counseling outcome research: Current trends and practical implications. *Journal of Counseling and Development, 74*, 590–9.

Sexton, T. L., & Whiston, S. C. (1996). Integrating counseling research and practice. *Journal of Counseling and Development, 74*, 588–9.

Schumacher, S., & McMillan, J. H. (1993). *Research in Education* (3rd ed.). New York: HarperCollins.

Smith, M. L., Glass, G. V., & Miller, T. (1980). *The Benefits of Psychotherapy*. Baltimore, MD: The John Hopkins University Press.

Snyder, C. R., & Ingrams, R. E. (Eds.). (2000). *Handbook of Psychological Change: Psychotherapy Processes and Practices for the 21st Century*. New York: John Wiley & Sons.

Strupp, H. H., Horowitz, L. M., & Lambert, M. J. (Eds.) (1997). *Measuring Patient Changes in Mood, Anxiety, and Personality Disorders: Toward a Core Battery*. Washington, DC: American Psychological Association.

Sullivan, R. K., & Mahalik, J. R. (2000). Increasing career self-efficacy for women: Evaluating a group intervention. *Journal of Counseling and Development, 78*, 54–62.

White, V. (2002). Personal communication.

Whiston, S. (1996). Accountability through action research: Research methods for practitioners. *Journal of Counseling and Development, 74*, 616–23.

RESOURCE W

Indirect Evidence: Methods for Evaluating the Presence of Nontherapy Explanations

NONCHANGE/NONTHERAPY POSSIBILITY

- Nonimprovement
  - A. Apparent changes are trivial.
  - B. Apparent changes are negative.
- Statistical artifacts
  - A. Apparent changes reflect measurement error.
  - B. Apparent changes reflect outlier or regression to the mean.
  - C. Apparent change is due to experimental error.
- Relational artifacts: Apparent changes are superficial attempts to please therapist/researcher.
- Apparent changes are result of client expectations or wishful thinking.
- Self-correction: Apparent changes reflect self-help and self-limiting easing of short-term or temporary problems.
- Apparent changes can be attributed to extratherapy life events (changes in relationships or work).
- Psychobiological factors: Apparent changes can be attributed to medication or herbal remedies or recovery from illness.
- Apparent changes can be attributed to reactive effects of research, including relation with research staff, altruism, etc.

STAYING WELL: GUIDELINES FOR RESPONSIBLE LIVING

⟱ *We often look at the world not as it is, but as we think it is. You are responsible for the life you create, regardless of the demands around you.*

OVERVIEW

GOALS

KEY CONCEPTS: A BALANCED LIFESTYLE WITH PROPORTION, NOT EQUITY
RULES FOR RESPONSIBLE LIVING
PRACTICAL REFLECTION 1: CLARIFYING YOUR VALUES
PRACTICAL REFLECTION 2: ASSESSING YOUR LOCUS OF CONTROL
PHYSICAL HEALTH
EMOTIONAL WELL-BEING
INTELLECTUAL ENRICHMENT
LIFE WORK SATISFACTION

SOCIAL EFFECTIVENESS
SPIRITUAL AWARENESS
PRACTICAL REFLECTION 3: YOUR LIFESTYLE ASSESSMENT SCORE
PRACTICAL REFLECTION 4: WELLNESS AND YOU: SETTING PERSONAL GOALS
PRACTICAL REFLECTION 5: THE CASE OF DARRYL AND COUNSELOR WELLNESS

SUMMARY AND PERSONAL INTEGRATION
PRACTICAL REFLECTION 6: INTEGRATION

REFERENCES
RESOURCES X AND Y

OVERVIEW

Awareness of wellness and a balanced lifestyle are critical to the success of your field experience, supervision in general, and your new professional life to come. Earlier in the book you looked at the importance of self-analysis. Understanding that you can only take your clients as far as you have gone yourself motivates you to continue self-reflection and maintenance of personal mental health. This chapter provides reflections and a lifestyle assessment to assist you with necessary skills and ideas for your own wellness.

GOALS

1. Understand that healthier helping professionals make for healthier clients.
2. Focus on a new model for integration of balance and wellness.
3. Be aware of wellness and its corresponding components.
4. Assess your personal wellness.
5. Set individual goals toward prevention and wellness.

KEY CONCEPTS: A BALANCED LIFESTYLE WITH PROPORTION, NOT EQUITY

When we started working on this chapter, the concept of integrating a balanced lifestyle into our personal and professional life was to be the main theme. As the chapter key concepts were formulated and I continued to think about your life as graduate students and my life as a mother, professor, and wife, the idea of balance becomes so difficult and complicated. Adding to this difficulty are the results from a study of mental health providers. Nearly one third of a large sample had experienced emotional exhaustion, poor sleep, chronic fatigue, loneliness, anxiety, or depression (Mahoney, 1997).

You want to have a balanced lifestyle, but trying to juggle all those pieces is so difficult and discouraging. Even the presumption of balance suggests equity and relatively equal parts on some level. However, if you were to create a formula for the amount of time you eat, intervene in life problems, play, sleep, study, and work, there would not be equal parts of time or energy. So perhaps there may be no such thing as a balanced lifestyle with equity of parts. If this is the case, the days of superwomen and supermen need to be banished. Instead you need to replace the old theory with a new model. This formula for responsible living achieves balance with proportional, not equitable, parts!

In class, I often use boxes that fit inside each other to demonstrate the idea of proportional parts. Once you know your most important values, then each box represents your values in order of priorities. Your most important value is shown and labeled using the biggest box. It is your foundation on which all other values stand. Value number two, represented by a smaller box, is important to your overall well-being, but it would not receive as much of your attention as value number one. This visual aid continues until I have at least five top values, and my boxes look like a stable tower with each value/box adding to the next!

Personal health and wellness are firmly founded on your own lifestyle. A classic piece of research stated that 20 percent of our lives are controlled by heredity, 19 percent by environment, and 10 percent by available health care (United States Public Health Service, 1979). Often you cannot control these percentages, but you can still make healthy choices around those things you cannot control. For example if there is heart disease in your family, you can still choose to eat heart healthy foods.

Burnout: Emotional and physical exhaustion due to excessive personal demands and depletion of resources.

That still leaves 51 percent of your life that you can shape by the choices you make! Listed in the next section are several guidelines for choosing to live wisely, responsibly, and intentionally. If you can live a healthy and balanced lifestyle, odds are you will not be at such risk for professional burnout and enjoy a long and satisfying career.

Try these rules to see if they are a good match for you. If not, there are other methods and perspectives for helping you create a sense of balance. It truly doesn't matter what model you adopt, as long as you are working on living healthfully.

Rules for Responsible Living

Rule #1: Clarify Your Values and Personal Expectations.   This must be accomplished with intentionality and the forethought of possible consequences. You have spent considerable time learning about intentional counseling. Intentional and responsible living is very similar. It is essential that you purposefully understand the why, the how, and the impact of the personal choices you make. Understanding these choices will make you a healthier counselor. If you know the why behind many of the personal choices you make, the odds are greater that you will better understand the decisions you make as a counselor!

A guess is that you don't spend as much time on your top values as you want and need! Remember in counseling we often tell clients that a value is something we must act upon. In other words, what we say must be congruent with what we do!

Practical Reflection 1: Clarifying Your Values

There are three interrelated aspects of this exercise. On a piece of paper write down the top five values in your life. Once you have listed them, determine the amount of time you spend with each of your top five values. Finally, use an asterisk to mark which value(s) you would like to devote more time to. Share your discoveries with your classmates.

Rule #2: Understand Your Personal Locus of Control.   In your counseling classes, many of you learned about Rotter's Locus of Control. This is useful information for our clients' well-being, but it can very easily generalize to your wellness, too. According to Rotter (1973), *locus of control* is the ability and belief about how much control you have over the events around you. Sometimes history and certain social events may determine your discourse and some of who you are, but you still have control over how you perceive events.

External locus of control suggests that others' opinions and influence, chance, and fate determine your destiny. *Internal locus of control* suggests that your own choices mainly determine your life and actions. Rotter believed you need both internal and external locus of controls. You need to have a ratio of three to one internal control to external control in order to have the skills necessary for healthy decision making (Brammer, Shostrum, & Abrego, 1992).

Those of you "who have a high degree of internality tend to be free thinkers, have the ability to critically evaluate the opinions of others and do not interject other points of view" (Neukrug, 1999, p. 12). If you can achieve high internal locus of control, there is evidence that you tend to be more respectful and have more empathy toward others with different points of view. Obviously the more internally controlled you are, the easier responsible living will be!

Practical Reflection 2: Assessing Your Locus of Control

Complete Rotter's Locus of Control Scale located in Resource X at the end of this chapter. Be as honest and spontaneous as you can. Try not to analyze each of the given paired statements too long! Score the scale according to the instructions to discover your total number of agreements. How might your results influence your ability to live responsibly and the manner in which you counsel others?

_____

_____

_____

_____

Wellness: An individualized experience using six dimensions to define wellness and balance: emotional, intellectual, physical, life work satisfaction, social, and spiritual.

Rule #3: Seek Understanding of These Personal Choices for Yourself.
One of the methods for understanding your personal choices is to examine the needed dimensions of wellness and your choices within each category. When you search the literature on wellness, typically many of the same categories are repeated with minor variations: physical, emotional, intellectual, occupational/life work, social, and spiritual (Adams, Bezner, & Steinhardt, 1997; Chapin & Russell-Chapin, 2003; Depken, 1994; Sackney, Noonan, & Miller, 2000; Thompson, 2001). As you read about the wellness dimensions, begin thinking about your personal wellness and lifestyle choices.

Physical Health

The dimension of physical health is essential to your personal wellness because it relates to your perceptions and expectations about physical health. Researchers have concluded that good or optimistic perceptions about physical health correlate positively with greater levels of actual physical activity (Fylkesnes & Forde, 1991; Rejeski et al., 2001). Remember if you don't have your physical health, overall wellness is often more difficult to obtain. However, the physical health dimension is not the biggest predictor of overall wellness. Can you guess which two dimensions hold the greatest predictive weight? Read on!

Emotional Well-Being

Being secure with who you are, the emotions you allow yourself to have, and your stated values are essential elements in overall wellness. *Emotional well-being* is multifaceted, but two major elements are strong self-esteem and a positive regard for who you are. Researchers have discovered that positive self-esteem is correlated to internal locus of control, physical activity, and a principle centeredness (Adams, Bezner, & Steinhardt, 1995). Your time in graduate school may sometimes work against this wellness dimension. Professors are constantly offering important feedback about your counseling skills and giving you earned grades. You must remember the feedback guidelines we wrote about in Chapter 1 of this book. Feedback is just about your skills not about you as a whole person!

Intellectual Enrichment

Intellectual enrichment is a fascinating category in the wellness formula. It is defined as your perception of just the right amount of intellectually stimulating information (Adams et al., 1997). Finding that "right amount" is important; researchers have found that too much or too little intellectual stimulation can negatively affect your health (Antonovsky, 1988.) This dimension is a difficult one for most graduate students. You must be careful not to experience the intellectual overload at the expense of the other wellness dimensions.

Life Work Satisfaction

Life work satisfaction is often associated with your choice of occupation as well. We prefer *life work satisfaction* because it denotes the idea of passion and satisfaction for all that your life entails (Chapin & Russell-Chapin, 2003). As you began to contemplate your graduate education, there was something about the helping professions that gave you pleasure and a sense of meaning and significance. Hopefully as you have learned new skills and techniques and gained more confidence as a person, your satisfaction and passion for life continues to grow.

Social Effectiveness

Social effectiveness or *social wellness* is one of the two dimensions that holds the highest predictive weight for overall wellness! You may have guessed correctly or perhaps you have experienced the need for a strong social network of friends and family. One definition of social effectiveness is the individual perception of having and providing support to self and

Practical Reflection 3: Your Lifestyle Assessment Score

Resource Y contains The Lifestyle Assessment Survey for you to take (Chapin & Russell-Chapin, 2003). You will be assessing the wellness dimensions described. Read the 60 wellness statements and honestly assess your current lifestyle. There are directions for administration and scoring. When you have calculated your results, write down your insights. Share your ideas with your classmates. You do not have to share your actual scores!

_____

_____

_____

_____

others (Adams et al., 1997). Studies have shown that social support is positively correlated with physical and psychological well-being (Manning & Fullerton, 1988)! The wellness dimension of social effectiveness is another difficult one to emphasize while in graduate school, because your time is filled with studying and other responsibilities. However, in the helping disciplines much of your graduate work may force you into groups and working teams. Some of your social support may actually be derived from your colleagues.

Spiritual Awareness

Spiritual awareness is emerging as the most fascinating dimension of wellness. It is the other wellness dimension that holds the highest predictive weight for overall wellness! There are many definitions of spiritual awareness, but the one that has the most empirical support is the positive perception and belief that every life has purpose, meaning, and significance (Crose, Nicholas, & Gobble, 1992). Researchers have discovered that a healthy spiritual life is associated with better physical and psychological health outcomes and overall well-being (Seybold & Hill, 2001; Zika & Chamberlain, 1992). Dr. Harold Koenig believes that our society is getting close to convincing people that religion and spirituality can help you stay healthy. Koenig and colleagues also write that those of you who are more spiritual experience greater well-being and life satisfaction, have less

---

Practical Reflection 4: Wellness and You: Setting Personal Goals

---

Using all the information you have gleaned from this chapter and your classmates, begin to formulate at least three individual wellness goals. Use your score from the Lifestyle Assessment Survey (LAS), the separate LAS statements and your reflections to set measureable goals. It could look something like:

I, _____ (your name), will begin to _____ (action) for at least _____ (time). I will evaluate my goal at the end of _____ (period of time). Be sure to share at least one of your goals with your classmates.

---

depression and anxiety, and are much less likely to commit suicide (Koenig, McCullough, & Larson, 2000).

Rule #4: Repeat and Share These Same Steps and Processes With Those Significant Others in Your Social System.   We live in a social world. Share your discoveries with significant others. This may include your partner, family members, special friends, work associates, and colleagues/students. The idea of listening to the feedback loop is essential in this phase of the model.

Once the feedback has been heard, a search for a consensus is needed, if the other person truly is a valued member of your life. You will begin to shape or balance your life and decisions by taking into account the resources, demands, and choices in your life.

Counselor impairment: A compromising condition due to a physical, emotional, or situational stressor that reduces the quality and effectiveness of counseling received by clients (Sheffield, 1998).

You are responsible for the life you create, inclusive of the demands around you! You also have a responsibility as a helping professional to maintain your own health for you, your family, and your clients (Iliffe & Steed, 2000; O'Halloran & Linton, 2000). Remember that what you say must be exactly what you do! If something is truly a value to you, then you need to act responsibly and consistently, if at all possible. By practicing a wellness philosophy, you increase your chances of not getting burned out from the stresses and demands involved in counseling. Burnout leads to counseling impairment, but a balanced lifestyle will decrease the odds that you will become impaired (Sheffield, 1998).

Practical Reflection 5: The Case of Darryl and Counselor Wellness

As you review the Case of Darryl, numerous scenarios come to mind concerning the possible wellness of Lori, the counselor. The first one you may want to discuss is the amount of time spent with this client. How could Lori keep herself well and maintain personal and professional boundaries? What are other concerns you may have about Darryl and living responsibly as a helping professional?

_____
_____
_____
_____

SUMMARY AND PERSONAL INTEGRATION

In Chapter 9, you were introduced to wellness constructs that could assist you in developing a personal wellness philosophy. A reframe of balanced living was presented to prevent counselor impairment.

- Rules for responsible living were provided.
- Six wellness dimensions were defined with corresponding reflections.
- A Lifestyle Assessment Survey was provided to assist you in developing wellness goals.

Practical Reflection 6: Integration

Which of the Chapter 9 ideas will help you the most in becoming a more balanced person and helping professional?

_____
_____
_____
_____

REFERENCES

Adams, T., Bezner, J., & Steinhardt, M. (1995). Principle-centeredness: A values clarification approach to wellness. *Measurement and Evaluation in Counseling and Development, 28,* 139–47.

Adams, T., Bezner, J., & Steinhardt, M. (1997). The conceptualization and measurement of perceived wellness: Integrating balance across and within dimensions. *American Journal of Health Promotion, 11,* 208–18.

Antonovosky, A. (1988). *Unraveling the mystery of health: How people manage stress and stay well.* San Francisco: Josey-Bass.

Brammer, L., Shostrum, E., & Abrego, P. (1992). *Therapeutic counseling and psychotherapy,* 6th ed. Englewood Cliffs, NJ: Prentice Hall.

Chapin, T., & Russell-Chapin, L. (2003). The lifestyle assessment survey: A self-report wellness survey. Manuscript under submission.

Crose, R., Nicholas D., & Gobble, D. (1992). Gender and wellness: A multidisciplinary systems model for counseling. *Journal of Counseling and Development, 71,* 149–56.

Depken, D. (1994). Wellness through the lens of gender: A paradigm shift. *Wellness Perspective, 10,* 54–69.

Fylkesnes, K., & Forde, O. (1991). The tromso study: Predictors of self-evaluated health—has society adopted the expanded health concept? *Social Science Medicine, 32,* 141–6.

Iliffe, G., & Steed, L. G. (2000). Exploring the counselor's experience of working with perpetrators of domestic violence. *Journal of Interpersonal Violence, 15,* 393–412.

Koenig, H., McCullough, M., & Larson, D. (2000). *The handbook of religion and health.* New York: Oxford University Press.

Mahoney, M. J. (1997). Psychotherapists' personal problems and self-care patterns. *Professional Psychology: Research and Practice, 28,* 14–16.

Manning, F., & Fullerton, T. (1988). Health and well-being in highly cohesive units of the US army. *Journal of Applied Social Psychology, 18,* 503–19.

Neukrug, E. (1999). *The world of the counselor: An introduction to the counseling profession.* Pacific Grove, Calif: Brooks/Cole.

O'Halloran, T. M., & Linton, J. M. (2000). Stress on the job: Self-care resources for counselors. *Journal of Mental Health Counseling, 22,* 354–64.

Rejeski, W. J., Shelton, B., Miller, M., Dunn, A. L., King, C. A., & Sallis, J. F. (2001). Mediators of increased physical activity and change in subjective well-being: Results from Activity Counseling Trials (ACT). *Journal of Health Psychology, 6,* 159–68.

Rotter, J. (1973). Internal/external locus of control scale. In J.P.Robinson and P.R. Shaver. (Eds.) *Measures of personality and social psychological attitudes,* 2nd ed. (pp. 227–34). Ann Arbor, Mich: Institute for Social Research, with permission from Elsevier.

Sackney, L., Noonan, B., & Miller, C. M. (2000). Leadership for educator wellness: An exploratory study. *International Journal of Leadership in Education, 3,* 41–56.

Seybold, K. S., & Hill, P. C. (2001). The role of religion and spirituality in mental and physical health. *Current Directions in Psychological Science, 10,* 21–4.

Sheffield, D. S. (1998). Counselor impairment: Moving toward a concise definition and protocol. *Journal of Humanistic Education and Development, 37,* 96–106.

Thompson, K. C. (2001). Dimensions of wellness and the health care matters program at Penn State. *Home Health Care Management and Practice, 13,* 308–11.

United States Public Health Service. (1979). *Preventable Mortality.* Washington, DC: US Department of Health Education and Welfare.

Zika, S., & Chamberlain, K. (1992). On the relation between meaning in life and psychological well-being. *British Journal of Psychology, 83,* 133–45.

RESOURCE X

Each statement has two choices. Select one of the given options.

Rotter's Locus of Control Scale*

1a. Children get into trouble because their parents punish
   them too much.   1a. ____
 b. The trouble with most children nowadays is that their
   parents are too easy with them.   b. ____
2a. Many of the unhappy things in people's lives are partly
   due to bad luck.   2a. ____
 b. People's misfortunes result from the mistakes they make.   b. ____
3a. One of the major reasons why we have wars is because
   people don't take enough interest in politics.   3a. ____
 b. There will always be wars, no matter how hard people
   try to prevent them.   b. ____
4a. In the long run people get the respect they deserve
   in this world.   4a. ____
 b. Unfortunately, an individual's worth often passes
   unrecognized no matter how hard he tries.   b. ____
5a. The idea that teachers are unfair to students is nonsense.   5a. ____
 b. Most students don't realize the extent to which their
   grades are influenced by accidental happenings.   b. ____
6a. Without the right breaks one cannot be an
   effective leader.   6a. ____
 b. Capable people who fail to become leaders have not
   taken advantage of their opportunities.   b. ____
7a. No matter how hard you try some people just
   don't like you.   7a. ____
 b. People who can't get others to like them don't
   understand how to get along with others.   b. ____
8a. Heredity plays the major role in determining
   one's personality.   8a. ____
 b. It is one's experiences in life which determine
   what they're like.   b. ____
9a. I have often found that what is going to happen
   will happen.   9a. ____

    b. Trusting to fate has never turned out as well for me
       as making a decision to take a definite course of action.   b. ____

10a. In the case of the well-prepared student there is rarely
      if ever such a thing as an unfair test.   10a. ____

    b. Many times exam questions tend to be so unrelated to
       course work that studying is really useless.   b. ____

11a. Becoming a success is a matter of hard work; luck has
      little or nothing to do with it.   11a. ____

    b. Getting a job depends mainly on being in the right place
       at the right time.   b. ____

12a. The average citizen can have an influence in
      government decisions.   12a. ____

    b. This world is run by the few people in power, and
       there is not much the little guy can do about it.   b. ____

13a. When I make plans, I am almost certain that I can
      make them work.   13a. ____

    b. It is not always wise to plan too far ahead because
       many things turn out to be a matter of good or
       bad fortune anyhow.   b. ____

14a. There are certain people who are just no good.   14a. ____
    b. There is some good in everybody.   b. ____

15a. In my case getting what I want has little or nothing
      to do with luck.   15a. ____

    b. Many times we might just as well decide what
       to do by flipping a coin.   b. ____

16a. Who gets to be the boss often depends on who was
      lucky enough to be in the right place first.   16a. ____

    b. Getting people to do the right thing depends upon
       ability, luck has little or nothing to do with it.   b. ____

17a. As far as world affairs are concerned, most of us are the
      victims of forces we can neither understand nor control.   17a. ____

    b. By taking an active part in political and social
       affairs the people can control world events.   b. ____

18a. Most people don't realize the extent to which
      their lives are controlled by accidental happenings.   18a. ____

    b. There really is no such thing as luck.   b. ____

19a. One should always be willing to admit mistakes.   19a. ____
    b. It is usually best to cover up one's mistakes.   b. ____

20a. It is hard to know whether or not a person really
      likes you.   20a. ____

    b. How many friends you have depends upon how
       nice a person you are.   b. ____

(continued)

RESOURCE X CONTINUED

21a. In the long run the bad things that happen to us are
balanced by the good ones.   21a. ____
   b. Most misfortunes are the result of lack of ability,
ignorance, laziness, or all three.   b. ____
22a. With enough effort we can wipe out political corruption. 22a. ____
   b. It is difficult for people to have much control over
the things politicians do in office.   b. ____
23a. Sometimes I can't understand how teachers arrive
at the grades they give.   23a. ____
   b. There is a direct connection between how hard
I study and the grades.   b. ____
24a. A good leader expects people to decide for themselves
what they should do.   24a. ____
   b. A good leader makes it clear to everybody what
their jobs are.   b. ____
25a. Many times I feel that I have little influence over
the things that happen to me.   25a. ____
   b. It is impossible for me to believe that chance or luck
plays an important role in my life.   b. ____
26a. People are lonely because they don't try to be
friendly.   26a. ____
   b. There's not much use in trying too hard to please
people, if they like you, they like you.   b. ____
27a. There is too much emphasis on athletics in high school.   27a. ____
   b. Team sports are an excellent way to build character.   b. ____
28a. What happens to me is my own doing.   28a. ____
   b. Sometimes I feel that I don't have enough control
over the direction my life is taking.   b. ____
29a. Most of the time I can't understand why politicians
behave the way they do.   29a. ____
   b. In the long run the people are responsible for bad
government on a national as well as on a local level.   b. ____

Score One Point for Each of the Following

2a, 3b, 4b, 5b, 6a, 7a, 9a, 10b, 11b, 12b, 13b, 15b, 16a, 17a, 18a, 20a, 21a,
22b, 23a, 25a, 26b, 28b, 29a

   A high score = external locus of control
   A low score = internal locus of control

I-E Scale Scoring Key

The I-E Scale is scored to indicate the total number of choices toward external locus of control. Read the following answers and check only those responses which agree with yours. Please note there are six filler items that are not scored. Total the number of agreements to determine your relative level of external locus of control. The smaller the total number of agreements, the less externally controlled you are.

_____	1.	_____	16. A
_____	2. A	_____	17. A
_____	3. B	_____	18. A
_____	4. B		19.
_____	5. B	_____	20. A
_____	6. A	_____	21. A
_____	7. A	_____	22. B
_____	8.	_____	23. A
_____	9. A		24.
_____	10. B	_____	25. A
_____	11. B	_____	26. B
_____	12. B		27.
_____	13. B	_____	28. B
_____	14.	_____	29. A
_____	15. B		

Total number of agreements or degree of external control: _____

RESOURCE Y

The Lifestyle Assessment Survey, Form C

Directions.   The following survey lists 60 statements reflective of a positive lifestyle. These statements are organized in six categories of wellness or optimal personal effectiveness. They include physical health, emotional well-being, intellectual enrichment, life work satisfaction, and spiritual awareness. For each section, read each statement and circle the number that best describes your behavior. Use the number code below. Then add the numbers you have circled to determine your score for that section. At the end of the survey, write the score from each section in the space provided and compute your total wellness score. The highest possible score is 300. Then interpret your wellness score with the key that is provided.

Number Code: 5 = Almost Always; 4 = Very Often; 3 = Often; 2 = Sometimes; 1 = Almost Never.

Physical Health Satisfaction

1. Complete 1/2 hour of daily aerobic exercise.   5 4 3 2 1
2. Eat a balanced diet from the four food groups.   5 4 3 2 1
3. Limit intake of caffeine, sugar, salt, and cholesterol.   5 4 3 2 1
4. Seek periodic health examinations.   5 4 3 2 1
5. Drive within traffic safety codes.   5 4 3 2 1
6. Avoid use of tobacco and other dangerous drugs.   5 4 3 2 1
7. Schedule time to relax each day.   5 4 3 2 1
8. Maintain ideal body weight.   5 4 3 2 1
9. Avoid drinking alcohol to intoxication.   5 4 3 2 1
10. Have deep and restful sleep.   5 4 3 2 1

Emotional Well-Being Effectiveness

11. Have a sense of humor and enjoy life.   5 4 3 2 1
12. Able to solve personal problems.   5 4 3 2 1
13. Enthusiastic about the future.   5 4 3 2 1
14. Accept responsibility for own actions.   5 4 3 2 1
15. Express feelings openly and genuinely.   5 4 3 2 1
16. Feel that you are loved.   5 4 3 2 1
17. Assertively communicate thoughts and feelings.   5 4 3 2 1
18. Able to avoid previous mistakes.   5 4 3 2 1
19. Comfortable with sexual behavior.   5 4 3 2 1
20. Accept and like yourself.   5 4 3 2 1

Intellectual Enrichment
Awareness

21. Attend cultural events (music, art, drama).   5 4 3 2 1
22. Read books, papers, or magazines.   5 4 3 2 1
23. Enjoy learning new information.   5 4 3 2 1
24. Have opportunities to be creative.   5 4 3 2 1
25. Interested in scientific breakthroughs.   5 4 3 2 1
26. Aware of social issues and current events.   5 4 3 2 1
27. Attend workshops or classes for personal benefit.   5 4 3 2 1
28. Exchange ideas and opinions with others.   5 4 3 2 1
29. Seek a variety of entertainment.   5 4 3 2 1
30. Enjoy science or historical museums.   5 4 3 2 1

Life Work

31. Enjoy my life work (school, work, or retirement).   5 4 3 2 1
32. Able to handle stress of life's work.   5 4 3 2 1
33. Motivated to make a meaningful contribution.   5 4 3 2 1
34. Feel a balance between life work and leisure.   5 4 3 2 1
35. Interested in life work.   5 4 3 2 1
36. Feel appreciated for my efforts.   5 4 3 2 1
37. Have plenty of opportunities to learn.   5 4 3 2 1
38. Feel challenged by my life's work.   5 4 3 2 1
39. Accept new or extra responsibilities.   5 4 3 2 1

40. Receive and accept feedback about life work.   5 4 3 2 1

Social

41. Enjoy intimate relationships.   5 4 3 2 1
42. Involved in the local community.   5 4 3 2 1
43. Provide help and support to others.   5 4 3 2 1
44. Enjoy friendships.   5 4 3 2 1
45. Comfortable with authority figures.   5 4 3 2 1
46. Accept others of different race, gender, or faith.   5 4 3 2 1
47. Enjoy family interactions.   5 4 3 2 1
48. Act to keep a clean natural environment.   5 4 3 2 1
49. Participate in group activities.   5 4 3 2 1
50. Take pride in personal environment.   5 4 3 2 1

Spiritual

51. Take time for quiet reflection or prayer.   5 4 3 2 1
52. Act out personal beliefs in daily life.   5 4 3 2 1
53. Act to help and care for others.   5 4 3 2 1
54. Respect the beliefs of others.   5 4 3 2 1
55. Search for meaning and value in life.   5 4 3 2 1
56. Support humanitarian causes.   5 4 3 2 1
57. Express values and beliefs to others.   5 4 3 2 1
58. Read inspirational materials.   5 4 3 2 1
59. Experience inner peace.   5 4 3 2 1
60. Follow a personal or group faith.   5 4 3 2 1

(continued)

RESOURCE Y CONTINUED

Results and Interpretation

SECTION	SCORE	RANGE	DESCRIPTION
Physical Health	_____	300–278	You have a healthy lifestyle and it shows!
Emotional Well-being	_____	277–248	Your efforts are paying off.
Intellectual Enrichment	_____	247–195	More effort and you will feel the difference.
Life Work Satisfaction	_____	194–168	You have the right idea. Keep at it.
Social Effectiveness	_____	<168	There's much you can do!
Spiritual Awareness	_____		
Total Wellness =	_____		

BECOMING A PROFESSIONAL HELPER: ADVOCACY FOR CLIENTS, SELF, AND THE PROFESSION

CHAPTER

10

> *The ultimate questions of psychotherapy are not a private matter—they represent a supreme responsibility. Carl G. Jung (1954)*

OVERVIEW

GOALS

KEY CONCEPTS: ADVOCACY AND ITS RELATIONSHIP TO THE TEN ESSENTIAL PRINCIPLES FOR HELPING PROFESSIONALS

ADVOCACY FOR THE CLIENT

ADVOCACY FOR SELF

ADVOCACY FOR THE PROFESSION
PRACTICAL REFLECTION 1: YOUR ADVOCACY EFFORTS

TEN ESSENTIAL CHAPTER PRINCIPLES FOR HELPING PROFESSIONALS
1. TRANSFERABLE SKILLS, ABILITIES, AND PRINCIPLES
PRACTICAL REFLECTION 2: LOOKING BACK AND COMPARING FEELINGS
2. CREATIVE INTERCHANGES THROUGH CORE INTERVIEWING SKILLS

3. THE PATH OF RIGHT ACTION
4. FLEXIBILITY IN GROWTH
5. ___ THE ENTIRE STORY
___ COMMUNICATION SKILLS
___ GEMENT AND THE WORLD
___
___ SED BEST PRACTICE
___ ND OTHERS
___ TION 3: WRITING NEW GOALS
___ FESSIONAL LIFE
10. ___ HERE AM I NOW AND WHERE DO I NEED TO GO?

SUMMARY AND PERSONAL INTEGRATION
PRACTICAL REFLECTION 4: INTEGRATION AND LESSONS LEARNED

REFERENCES
RESOURCE Z

OVERVIEW

Advocacy is the central theme of this chapter, demonstrating that you must advocate for your clients, yourself, and the helping professions. A review of the book chapters is provided, summarizing the essential variables for a successful field experience and how advocacy is an integral part of that experience. A planning program and goal setting for continuing education, further supervision, and advocacy for the profession is included.

GOALS

1. Advocate for your clients, self, and the profession as an integral component of being a professional helper.
2. Review the key components necessary for you to continue having a successful counseling career.
3. Understand the importance of personal and professional advocacy.
4. Realize the benefits of practicing healthy risk management.
5. Set new goals at the end of your field experience.

KEY CONCEPTS: ADVOCACY AND ITS RELATIONSHIP TO THE TEN ESSENTIAL PRINCIPLES FOR HELPING PROFESSIONALS

As you complete your practicum and internship, you must congratulate yourself for your continued growth and risk taking! Look back and be amazed at all you and your clients have achieved.

Advocacy: The art of promoting and supporting the efforts and skills of a person, cause, or profession.

Much of what you accomplished came about because of advocacy efforts. *Advocacy* is offering support and assistance promoting a cause, skills, an individual, and/or an organization. This advocacy work may have been disguised in different ways, but each played an important part in the success of your clients, you, and your profession.

ADVOCACY FOR THE CLIENT

As we have stated, often clients enter into your life in a vulnerable state. Their past efforts at resolving concerns may have been unsuccessful. Once again it is your ethical and professional responsibility to assist clients in overcoming obstacles, fears, and injustices.

That is only the first step, and it may be the least difficult to accomplish. It is not enough to teach individual clients new coping skills. Also you need to move into the community and work upstream to educate, teach, and prevent oppression and racism and all other dimensions of diversity.

ADVOCACY FOR SELF

Promotion for self is difficult to do, because most helping professionals are very altruistic by nature. You may have been taught that advocating may be equivalent to bragging or selfishness. But you will learn that if you don't advocate for yourself, often no one else will. Assertiveness and colleagueship are essential features of advocating for oneself. A wonderful definition of assertiveness includes the concept of mutual respect. You respect yourself enough to share your thoughts, feelings, and behaviors with others in a mutually respectful manner. You teach your clients the importance of healthy communication; it is time to practice what you preach!

It is essential that you let others in the community know what you can do as a professional helper. Don't be afraid to sell your skills and outcomes. Recently a student of mine named Maria wanted to work in a hospital setting. Her credentials and skills were outstanding, but she did not even receive an initial interview. I encouraged Maria to ask for an appointment to share with the interviewer what her skills could do for that particular program. Even if she was not hired, that same supervisor would know more about her skills than before. Maria was brave enough to call again and the appointment was scheduled, not as a job interview but as an information giving session. The reluctant supervisor listened intently. I strongly encouraged Maria to point out her strengths. She had training in counseling diverse populations, was multilingual, and had completed her thesis on eating disorders and adolescence.

Maria stated that the interviewer was stunned when she was finished stating how Maria could make a difference in this program. Maria did not get that job, but in a month another position opened up, and Maria was hired! Advocating for self is not bragging, it is respectfully educating others about you, your skills, and the profession!

Another component of advocacy for self is to remember the value of supervision and listening to critiques. The more trusting feedback you can receive, the more skilled you become. The same is true when your colleagues seek you out in assistance. All of us find ourselves working in oppressive situations in our jobs from time to time. Advocating also means helping others with job-related stressors.

Practical Reflection 1: Your Advocacy Efforts

What are you doing now or can you do to promote the needs of your clients, yourself, and the profession? Be specific.

_____

_____

_____

_____

ADVOCACY FOR THE PROFESSION

You are beginning to understand how advocating for your clients and self is an indirect way of advocating for your profession. There are many reasons why you need to advocate for your profession, but current times are calling for budget cuts in our local communities, the state, and nation. Counseling centers, community centers, and social service programs have experienced budget cuts to deal with deficits in spending. How can you not sell yourself and your agency to those around you during these times?

In Chapter 7, you were strongly encouraged to join professional organizations. This is another natural way to be active in necessary lobbying efforts that are constantly underway to ensure that mental health services continue and that you remain with updated skills.

As you review the summary of chapters, think about how each chapter and the material presented can assist you in your advocacy efforts. In short, be smart and always think how you can advocate for the clients, yourself, and the profession!

TEN ESSENTIAL CHAPTER PRINCIPLES FOR HELPING PROFESSIONALS

1. Transferable Skills, Abilities, and Principles

First, as you begin to complete your practicum and internship experience, there are many skills, abilities, and principles for you to integrate and practice. You might be feeling overwhelmed again, as you leave your

---

Practical Reflection 2: Looking Back and Comparing Feelings

How are these feelings about completing your graduate education similar and different from those when you first started your practicum and internship?

_____

_____

_____

_____

---

structured graduate education. This is your chance to review and remember all that you have learned in this clinical experience.

At the beginning of this book you were asked to accept your fears and insecurities and turn them into facilitative energy to help you move forward. You will need to use that same structure again to ease your way through this next transition . . . actually graduating and transitioning into a job as a certified and soon licensed counseling professional!

Go back through Chapter 1, "Turning Theory Into Practice: Abilities Needed to Grow." Review your practical reflections and necessary abilities. These will assist you in generalizing those ideas and strategies to this new and different stage in your life. This skill of generalizing from one situation to another relevant situation is often exactly what we ask our clients to do!

2. Creative Interchanges Through Core Interviewing Skills

In Chapter 2, "Listening to Tapes and Analyzing Cases: Microcounseling Supervision," you were introduced to the Microcounseling Supervision Model (MSM). You have reviewed and practiced many of the necessary micro- and macrocounseling communication skills as you interviewed all your clients. You must continue practicing those skills, and soon they will become very natural components of your personality and skill base. You will use those same skills in counseling and in everyday living. Those core interviewing skills will assist you in having creative interchanges with everyone you meet. What a bonus for you and those around you!

3. The Path of Right Action

Chapter 3 introduced you to "Becoming Effective as a Supervisee: The Influence of Placement Setting." Discussions of placement sites and their influence were presented, and the qualities of an effective supervisee were discussed. You will continue to use the skills as you set up new supervision schedules in your next counseling position.

Your major task now in the rank of counseling professional will be to make wise and ethical decisions and try to consistently take the path of right action. The term *right action* encompasses almost everything we do as counselors: human welfare, social justice, and counseling competency.

4. Flexibility in Growth

In Chapter 4, "Continuing Self Improvement: Major Categories of Supervision Models," you were introduced to the three main supervision models: developmental, integrated, and theoretical specific. As you continue to grow, so will your desired supervision model and needs.

Continue to be flexible. Continue to engage in your own outcome research and be sure to keep up with the latest research on supervision. New research will challenge you to stretch and try new ideas. For example, Ray and Altekruse (2000) conducted group supervision research. Their results may have great implications on how supervision is conducted; they found that group supervision is not only complementary to individual supervision, but that it may be exchanged for individual supervision! Change in you and change in the profession will always keep you active and challenged!

5. Telling the Entire Story

Chapter 5, "Conceptualizing the Client: Diagnosis and Related Issues," introduced you to client conceptualization, related treatment, and diagnosis. You learned the importance of multiaxial diagnosis using the DSM-IV-TR and that each of the five axes gave you a clear picture of the client's concerns. As it is in counseling, looking at the entire picture adds clarity and depth. This skill, too, can generalize to your life. Make sure that you are looking at the big picture of your new professional counseling life and your personal life. Get all the supervision and support to make it work well.

6. Universal Communication Skills

"Becoming a Culturally Competent Helping Professional: Appreciation of Diversity" was the theme of Chapter 6. You were introduced to muticultural models and cultural identity development. Remember that the profession of counseling as an organized and standardized organization is still very young throughout the world, but the function of counseling transcends years and years of organizations and cultures. In a study by Bond and co-workers, (2001), who researched the nature of counseling in fifteen countries on every continent, results emphasized that counseling is a socially constructed mechanism. In many of these countries the term *counseling* was not even recognized, but what translated through the languages were universal and facilitative communication skills that help others to solve relevant cultural problems. The universal skills were those we tend to label as active listening, empathy, and self-empowering skills!

The results of this research are extremely important for you as a beginning helping professional. You cannot impose your cultural values on others, but you can listen and work within the client's framework.

7. Risk Management and the World of Counseling

In Chapter 7, "Working with Ethics, Laws, and Professionalism: Best Practice Standards," you read about the ethical guidelines that assist us professionally. Landmark case law and skills necessary to be successful in counseling practice, such as record keeping, case notes, and referral procedures, were also emphasized. The HIPAA regulations were discussed with practical suggestions for implementation.

You are beginning to understand that it is your job as a counselor to advocate for all your clients. As counselors and helping professionals, you continually strive to affect human welfare in a positive manner (Montgomery, Cupit, & Wimberley, 1999). With advocacy and counseling come risks. That is why you must continue to be supervised, maintain your professional licenses and certifications, hold memberships in professional organizations, and obtain excellent malpractice insurance. In a recent survey exploring professional issues and personal experiences related to malpractice, the authors were surprised that the threat of malpractice actually has resulted in better informed helping professionals and increased attention to best practice activities (Montgomery et al., 1999).

As Carl Jung (1954) so aptly stated, "Small and invisible as the contribution may be, it is still a magnum opus . . . . The ultimate questions of psychotherapy are not a private matter—they represent a supreme responsibility."

8. Evidence-Based Best Practice

Chapter 8, "Counseling Research Outcomes: Discovering What Works," offered material about the efficacy of counseling. You were encouraged to ask three essential questions about your counseling effectiveness. You were also asked to make a commitment to conducting your own personal research to advance the field of counseling. Different research designs were reviewed and explored. Evaluating your individual and group counseling sessions, skills, counseling styles, and programs on a consistent basis was encouraged and recommended.

9. Helping Self and Others

Chapter 9, "Staying Well: Guidelines for Responsible Living" presented information about the importance of keeping well as a helping professional. The chapter offered you an opportunity to consider balance from a viewpoint of proportion as opposed to equity. You were able to assess your wellness lifestyle and set several personal wellness goals.

One of many things you can do to ensure your professional balance is to join professional associations that will assist you in keeping in touch with the latest advances in your specialties or in the counseling profession in general. Another excellent way to ensure professional health is to present or teach the material that you believe others need to know. In other words, be an active member of the profession. As you network with others, your knowledge seems to grow exponentially. Remaining current by continuing education, attending conferences, and reading professional journals is vital to your wellness.

Practical Reflection 3: Writing New Goals for Your Professional Life

Review your old goals and evaluate your success. If all your goals were achieved, select three new measurable goals to assist you in this transition between ending your graduate career and beginning a new job. You may want to continue one of your previous goals as well.

_____

_____

_____

_____

Several times throughout this text you had an opportunity to assess your counseling skills, supervision style, and wellness philosophy. You were asked to set personal goals for this class and for creating a balanced lifestyle. Go back to those goals to reassess how you are doing in your counseling goals and personal life. After reviewing the goals, it may be time to set new goals.

10. Where Am I Now and Where Do I Need to Go?

In Chapter 10, "Becoming a Professional Helper: Advocacy for Clients, Self, and the Profession," you reviewed all ten chapters in this text. Chapter 10 encourages you to be an advocate for your clients, yourself, and the counseling profession. *Advocacy* is to promote and move forward a certain effort, person, or organization. We are using the term here to request that you assert your thoughts, actions, and deeds concerning the complementary and unique skills that professional helpers demonstrate. There are many advocacy resources available, but you must recognize that you and your skills as a professional counselor are some of the best resources offered for you, your clients, and the general population (Kiselica & Robinson, 2001).

Each helping discipline has guidelines and plans for advocating for clients, individuals, and the profession. A professional counseling organization that promotes and advocates for the profession is Chi Sigma Iota, the international counseling honorary. During the past few years, leaders in Chi Sigma Iota have been identifying components of advocacy and presenting these to members of the counseling professions. Resource Z lists advocacy themes from Chi Sigma Iota. You may also want to locate advocacy resources on the web at http://www.csi-net.org and http://www.counseling. org/government_relations/pdfs/counselor.

As you look over your practicum and internship, reflect on all that you have gained. Remember your fears, insecurities, and joys, and those of your clients. Your counseling career is just beginning, and you will continue to grow with every new client. As you grow, so does the counseling profession. Continue to be flexible and find "within the narrative of psychological healing a place for tools plundered from related disciplines." (Simon, 2002, p.45).

We hope your field experience journey has been an adventure filled with joys, challenges, and fears. You have entered an exciting profession. May it bring you a lifetime of satisfaction and growth! Be sure to fill out the evaluation at the end of this book giving us feedback about your journey!

Practical Reflection #4: Integration and Lessons Learned

What has been the biggest lesson you have learned during your field experiences? Was it an advocacy lesson for your client, yourself, or the profession? Share with your colleagues as a closing exercise.

_____

_____

_____

_____

SUMMARY AND PERSONAL INTEGRATION

Chapter 10 began the integration efforts from your practicum and internship experiences.

- Chapters 1 through 10 were summarized.
- You were requested to make new goals for your future.
- The importance of advocating and being smart for your client, yourself, and the profession was emphasized.

REFERENCES

Bond, T., Courtland, L., Lowe, A., Malayapillay, M., Wheeler, S., Banks, A., Kurdt, K., Mercado, M., & Smiley, E. (2001). The nature of counselling: An investigation of counselling activity in selected countries. *International Journal for the Advancement of Counselling, 23,* 245–260.

Jung, C. G. (1954). *The practice of psychotherapy,* vol. 16. London: Routledge & Kegan Paul.

Kiselica, M., & Robinson, M. (2001). Bringing advocacy counseling to life: The history, issues, and human drama of social justice in counseling. *Journal of Counseling and Development, 79,* 387–97.

Montgomery, L. M., Cupit, B. E., & Wimberlely, T. K. (1999). Complaints, malpractice, and risk management: Professional issues and personal experiences. *Professional Psychology: Research and Practice, 30,* 402–10.

Ray, D., & Altekruse, M. (2000). Effectiveness of group supervision versus combined group and individual supervision. *Counselor Education and Supervision, 40,* 19–30.

Simon, R. (2002, June). The larger story. *Psychotherapy Networker, 45–46.* Washington, D.C.

RESOURCE Z

Chi Sigma Iota Advocacy Themes

Theme A: Counselor Education

GOAL: To ensure that all counselor education students graduate with a clear identity and sense of pride as professional counselors.

Theme B: Intra-professional Relations

GOAL: To develop and implement a unified, collaborative advocacy plan for the advancement of counselors and those whom they serve.

Theme C: Marketplace Recognition

GOAL: To ensure that professional counselors in all settings are suitably compensated for their services and free to provide service to the public within all areas of their competence.

Theme D: Inter-professional Issues

GOAL: To establish collaborative working relationships with other organizations, groups, and disciplines on matters of mutual interest and concern to achieve our advocacy goals for both counselors and their clients.

Theme E: Research

GOAL: To promote professional counselors and the services they provide based on scientifically sound research.

Name Index

Abrego, P., 223
Adams, T., 224–226
Altekruse, M., 242
American Counseling Association, 163, 177
American Psychiatric Association, 104, 112, 121
American Psychological Association, 163
Antonovsky, A., 225
Arredondo, P., 129–132
Ashen, A., 113, 115
Asner, K. K., 212
Authur, G. L., 164, 170, 171

Bailey, A., 3
Baird, B. N., 164–165
Baker, S. B., 20
Banks, A., 243
Barks, C., xix, xx
Barlow, D. H., 208, 213
Basham, R., 212
Bathchelder, D., 138
Beauchamp, T. L., 164
Belwood, M. F., 211
Berger, S., 137
Bergman, J. S., 110
Bernard, J. M., 91–93, 95
Bezner, J., 224–225
Blanchard, J. M., 50
Bond, T., 243
Borders, L. D., 93
Boyer, E. L., 215–216
Brammer, L., 223

Callanan, P., 165
Carrol, M., 88
Cattani-Thompson, K., 209
Chamberlain, K., 226
Chapin, T., 224–226
Childress, J. F., 164
Cook, D. A., 136
Corey, G., 93, 165
Corey, M., 165
Courtland, L., 243
Crose, R., 226
Cupit, B. E., 243
Curtis, R. C., 5

Daniels, T., 20
Delworth, U., 50, 89, 95
Depken, D., 224
Dimick, K. M., 68
Doehrmann, M., 95
Dunn, A. L., 224

Egan, G., 108
Elliot, R., 209–212
Ellis, A., 92
Eysenck, H., 209

Falvey, J. E., 170–171
Forde, O., 224
Friedlander, M. L., 50, 96
Fullerton, T., 226
Fylkesnes, K., 224

Ginter, G., 110–113, 117
Glass, G. V., 209

Glossoff, H. L., 171
Gobble, D., 226
Goodyear, R. K., 91–93, 96
Greenberg, L. S., 209

Haaga, D. A., 209
Haase, R., 19
Hackney, H. L., 70, 96
Halgin, R. P., 95
Hathaway, S. R., 110
Hayes, S. C., 208, 213
Haynes, R., 93
Helms, J. E., 129, 136–137
Heppner, P. P., 209
Herlihy, B., 171
Hershey, P., 50
Hill, P. C., 226
Holloway, E., 88
Horowitz, L. M., 209

Iliffe, G., 227
Ingrams, R. E., 208
Ivey, A., 9–10, 19, 21, 94, 107, 113, 114,
    130, 131
Ivey, M., 21, 94, 107, 113–114, 130

Jaffee v. Redmond, 170
Johnson, D., 50
Jung, C. G., 4, 237, 243

Kadushin, A., 88
Kagan, N., 93
Kaplan, D., 164
Keith-Spiegel, P., 164
Kenny, M., 168
King, C. A., 224
King, M., 70
Kiselica, M., 245
Kivlighan, D. M., 210
Kjos, D., 109
Koenig, H., 226–227
Koocher, G., 164
Kopala, L. A., 213
Kottler, J., 130
Krause, F. H., 68
Kurdt, K., 243
Kwan, K. K., 129, 132

Lambert, M. J., 19, 208–209
Landany, M., 51
Larson, D., 227

Leddick, G. R., 93
Linton, J. M., 227
Lowe, A., 243
Lundervold, D. A., 211

Mace, C., 208–209, 213
Magnuson, S., 213
Mahalik, J. R., 212
Mahoney, M. J., 221
Malayapillay, M., 243
Manning, F., 226
Marotta, S., 51, 212
McCullough, M., 227
McDavis, R. J., 129, 131–132
McKinley, J. C., 110
McMillan, J. H., 213
McNeill, B., 50, 89
Mercado, M., 243
Miller, C., 19–20
Miller, C. M., 224
Miller, M., 224
Miller, T., 209
Millon, T., 110
Mitchell, R. W., 166
Montgomery, L. M., 243
Moorey, S., 209, 213
Morrill, W., 19, 20
Moulton, P., 93
Moursand, J., 168
Muse-Burke, J. 51

National Association of Social Workers,
    163
National Organization of Human Service
    Professionals, 163
Nelson-Gray, R. O., 208, 213
Neukrug, E., 211, 213, 223
Nicholas, D., 226
Noonan, B., 224
Norcross, J. C., 95
Norem, K., 213
Normington, C., 19
Nye, S., 70
Nwachuku, U. T., 131

Ogles, B. M., 19
O'Halloran, T. M., 227
Olk, M., 96

Patterson, D., 212
Pederson, P., 130, 136

Ray, D., 242
Rejeski, W. J., 224
Roberts, B., 209
Robinson, M., 245
Rogers, C., 7, 92
Rotter, J., 223
Russell-Chapin, L. A., 20, 137–140, 224, 225, 226
Russo, J. R., 51

Sackney, L., 224
Sallis, J. F., 224
Sanders-Thompson, V., 146
Schmidt, A., xiii
Schumacher, S., 213
Schuyler, D., 168
Scissons, E. H., 20
Sexton, T., 210, 215
Seybold, K. S., 226
Sheffield, D. J., 227
Shelton, B., 224
Sherman, N. E., 20, 53
Shostrum, E., 223
Simon, R., 245
Smart, D., 114
Smart, J., 114
Smiley, E., 243
Smith, M. L., 209
Snyder, C. R., 208
Spence, E. B., 171
Steed, L. G., 227
Steinhardt, N., 224–226
Stiles, W. B., 209

Stoltenberg, C. D., 50, 89, 95, 177
Stoner, C., 137–140
Strupp, H. H., 209
Sue, D., 130
Sue, D. W., 129, 130–132
Sullivan, R. K., 212
Suzuki, M., 213
Swanson, C. D., 164, 170–171
Sweitzer, H. F., 70

Tarasoff v. Regents of the University of California, 169
Thompson, K. C., 224
Tomes, J. T., 167

Uhlemann, M., 20
United States Department of Health and Human Services, 111
United States Public Health Service, 222

Wampold, B. E., 210
Ward, L. G., 50
Warner, E., 138
Wheeler, S., 243
Whiston, S., 208, 215
White, V., 207
Wilcoxen, A. S., 213
Wimberely, T. K., 243
Woods, P. J., 92

Zika, S., 226
Zuckerman, E., 165

Subject Index

Activating event, 137
Advocacy, 238–240
    clients, 238
    definition, 238
    profession, 240
    self, 239
American Counseling Association, 163, 172

Case notes, 166–167
    health insurance portability accountability act (HIPAA), 166–168
    record keeping, 166
Case of Darryl
    preface, xvii
    transcript, 140–146
Case of Rachel, 37
    case conceptualization, 223–228
    narrative case presentation example, 218–223
    preface, xv
    supervision, 94–96
    transcript, 22–26
Case of Stephen, 114
    preface, xvii
    transcript, 56–58, 144–148
Case law, 169–171
    definition, 169
    duty to warn–Tarasoff, 169
    privilege communication–Jaffee, 170–171
Case presentation, 29, 117–118
Cautiousness, 106–107
Change, 12, 209

Chi Sigma Iota, 245
    resource Z, Chi Sigma Iota advocacy themes, 247
Code of Ethics for the Helping Professionals, 165
Conceptualization strategies, 107–109
    case of Rachel, 120–122
    developmental assessment, 113–116
    diagnostic and statistical manual of mental disorders, 108, 109–113
    stages of the counseling interview, 107–108
    telling the entire story, 242
Confidentiality, 105
    colleges and universities, 61
    community agencies, 63–64
    definition, 164
    exception to confidentiality, 170
    hospital-based treatment programs, 67
    private practice, 66
    school, 55
Counseling Interview Rating Form (CIRF), 19
    counseling skills baseline, 30
    creation of, 20
    definition, 58
    resource C, blank CIRF, 41–42
    scoring, 27
    uses, 28–29
Counselor impairment, 227
    burnout, 222
    definition, 222
Countertransference issues, 14
    definition, 14

Defensiveness, 12
Development style, 113–116
    concrete orientation, 114
    dialectic-systemic orientation, 115
    formal-operational orientation, 114
    sensorimotor orientation, 114
    triadic imagery method, 115
Diagnosis
    case conceptualization, 104–107
    definition, 105
Duty to warn, 169

Ethics, 162–163
    American Counseling Association, 163
    ethical behaviors and practice, 164–165
    ethical guidelines, 165
    National Organization of Human
        Service Professionals, 163
    path of right action, 242
    social justice, 162
Evaluation, 70–71
    program, 212–213
Evidence base counseling, 208
    counseling effectiveness and change,
        209–210
    definition, 210
    outcome research, 210–214

Fears and concerns, 5
Feedback
    constructive feedback, 6–7
    corrective feedback, 7
    definition, 6
    preface, xiv

Goals setting
    areas for growth and development, 4–6
    goals for Rachel, 121–122
    personal goals, 6
    preface, xiii
    treatment plans, 116–117
    wellness, 227
Global assessment of functioning, 112
    axis V, 112
    definition, 112
Guest house, preface, xix

Health Insurance Portability and
    Accountability Act (HIPAA),
    166–167
    definition, 167

Immediacy in counseling, 36
Informed consent, 164
    definition, 164
Intentionality, 34
    definition, 21
International classification of diseases,
    111–112
Interpersonal process recall, 93–94

Jaffee v. Redmond, 170

Microcounseling Associates, Inc.,
    preface, xvi
Microcounseling skills
    creative interchanges, 241
    definition, 19
    effectiveness, 20
Microcounseling Supervision Model, 18–28
    classifying skills with mastery, 21–22
    definition, 20
    processing supervisory needs, 26–27
    reviewing skills with intention, 20
Multiaxial diagnosis, 109
    axis I, 109–110
    axis II, 110–111
    axis III, 111–112
    axis IV, 112
    axis V, 112
Multicultural competency standards, 132
    attitudes and belief guidelines, 132–133
    definition, 132
    knowledge guidelines, 133–135
    skills guidelines, 135
Multicultural counseling, 132
    stages, 130
    universal communication skills, 242
Multicultural issues
    preface, xiv
    components, 9
    cross-cultural dimensions, 130–131
    identity, 132
    racial development phases, 135–137

National Association of Social Workers,
    163
National Organization of Human Service
    Professionals, 163

Outcome research, 209–214
    definition, 209
    descriptive research, 211

meta analysis, 213
   qualitative designs, 213–214
   quantitative designs, 211–212
Outcome research theoretical models,
   214–216
   research practitioner, 214
   scientist practitioner, 214–215
   teacher scholar, 215–216

Perceptual switch, 139
Personal counseling, 13
Personal strengths, 10–11
Personality disorders, 110–111
   definition, 110
Placement settings
   colleges and universities, 59–61
   community agencies, 61–64
   hospital-based treatment programs,
     66–67
   private practice, 64–66
   school settings, 53–55
Power, 8–9
Praxis, preface, xvi, 3
Privileged communication, 170
   definition, 171
Professionalism, 171, 243
   definition, 172
   professional behaviors, 172
   risk management, 243
Professional organizations, 172–173
   American Counseling Association,
     163, 172
   American Mental Health Counseling
     Association, 172
   American Psychological Association,
     172
   American School Counselor
     Association, 172
   Association for Multicultural
     Counseling and Development, 172
   Association of Specialists in Group
     Work, 172
   British Association for Counselling
     and Psychotherapy, 172
   Canadian Psychological Association,
     172
   National Association for Social
     Workers, 163, 172
   National Organization for Human
     Service Educators, 163
   Resource U, Web addresses, 176

Qualitative research, 213–214
   behavioral observations, 213
   definition, 213
Quantitative research, 211–212
   definition, 211
   single case design, 211–212

Racial identity models, 136
   people of color, 136
   white, 136
   Helm's interactional process, 136–137
Referrals, 168–169
Release of information, 170
   definition, 170
Resistance, 12
Resources for the field
   resource A, Glossary of CIRF Skills,
     33–37
   resource B, Microskill Classification of
     the Case of Rachel, 38–40
   resource C, Blank CIRF, 41–42
   resource D, Authors' Quantification of
     CIRF for the Case of Rachel,
     43–45
   resource E, Blank CIRF, Establishing
     a Baseline, 46–47
   resource F, Supervisory Styles
     Inventory, 73–74
   resource G, Completed CIRF for the
     Case of Stephen, 75–77
   resource H, Student Practicum/
     Internship Agreement, 78
   resource I, Practicum/Internship
     Contract, 79–80
   resource J, Weekly Log, 81
   resource K, Client Informed
     Consent, 82
   resource L, Client Release Form, 83
   resource M, Site Supervisor's
     Evaluation of Student Counselor's
     Performance, 84–86
   resource N, Microcounseling Skills
     Used in Other Theories, 99
   resource O, Supervisee Perception of
     Supervision, 100–102
   resource P, Microskills Hierarchy, 124
   resource Q, Case Presentation Outline
     Guide, 125
   resource R, Blank CIRF, 149–150
   resource S, Completed CIRF for the
     Case of Darryl, 151–154

Resources for the field (continued)
    resource T, Skill Identification for the
        Case of Darryl, 155–160
    resource U, Web addresses for
        Professional Organizations and
        Codes of Ethics, 176
    resource V, ACA Code of Ethics,
        177–206
    resource W, Indirect evidence:
        Methods for evaluating the
        presence of nontherapy
        explanations, 219
    resource X, Rotter's Locus of Control,
        230–233
    resource Y, The Lifestyle Assessment
        Survey, 234–236
    resource Z, Chi Sigma Iota Advocacy
        Themes, 247
Respect, 7
Responsible living, 222–228
    clarifying values, 222–223
    locus of control, 223
Risk-taking, 4
    definition, 4

Scheduling counseling appointments, 12
Simulation
    albatross, 137–140

Social justice, 162
    national association of social
        workers, 163
Supervision
    definition, 8, 49, 88
    developmental stages, 50
    flexibility, 242
    functions, 88
    role, 89
    style, 50
Supervision models
    developmental, 89–90
    integrated, 90–92
    theoretical specific, 92

Tarasoff v. Regents of the University of
    California, 169
    case law, 169–171
Transference issues, 13–14
    definition, 14

Wellness, 224–227
    definition, 224
    emotional well-being, 225
    intellectual enrichment, 225
    life work satisfaction, 225
    social effectiveness, 225–226
    spiritual awareness, 226